Little Madam

Understanding And Parenting Your Girl Child With ADHD

By

Nancy S. Henders

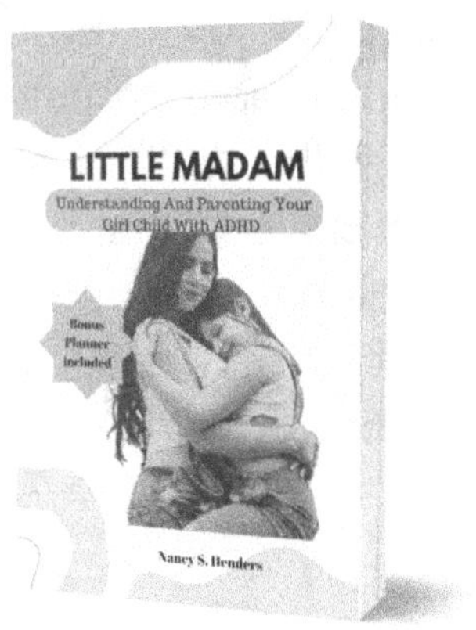

Understanding and Parenting Your Girl Child with ADHD

Table of Contents

Introduction

Once upon a time, in a bustling neighborhood, there lived a bright and spirited girl named Maya. From a young age, Maya exhibited a natural inclination towards taking charge and organizing activities. Whether it was planning elaborate games with her friends or spearheading school projects, Maya had a knack for leadership. However, her assertiveness often led to her being labeled as "bossy" by both peers and adults alike.

Maya's journey with ADHD began to unfold as she entered elementary school. While her peers struggled to sit still and focus, She found herself constantly fidgeting and daydreaming. She had a hard time following instructions and staying on task, which often resulted in incomplete assignments and forgotten responsibilities. Despite her best efforts, Maya's academic performance suffered, and she began to feel frustrated and misunderstood.

As Maya's symptoms became more pronounced, so did the criticism from others. Teachers would reprimand her for being disruptive in class, while classmates would tease her for being "bossy" and controlling. Maya's confidence began to wane, and she started to doubt her abilities. She wondered why she couldn't be like the other kids, effortlessly blending in and following the rules.

One day, Maya's parents decided to seek professional help to understand her behavior better. After consulting with a pediatrician and undergoing a comprehensive evaluation, Maya was diagnosed with ADHD. While the diagnosis initially came as a shock to Maya and her family, it also brought a sense of relief and clarity. Finally, they had an explanation for Maya's struggles and could start exploring strategies to support her.

The strategies that Maya and her parents used are explored in this book. This is a guide for parents who are navigating the journey of raising a daughter with attention-deficit hyperactivity disorder (ADHD). In these pages, we will explore the unique challenges and opportunities that come with parenting a girl with ADHD, offering insights, strategies, and support to help you and your daughter thrive.

The Invisible Struggle

Girls with ADHD often face distinct challenges that differ from those experienced by boys with the same condition. While boys with ADHD may exhibit more externalizing behaviors such as hyperactivity and impulsivity, girls with ADHD tend to display internalizing symptoms such as inattention, disorganization, and emotional dysregulation. As a result, girls with ADHD are more likely to go undiagnosed or misdiagnosed, leading to delays in receiving appropriate support and intervention.

The underdiagnosis of ADHD in girls can be attributed to various factors, including societal expectations, gender biases, and the presentation of symptoms. Girls with ADHD are often labeled as "daydreamers," "spacey," or "quiet," which may mask their underlying struggles with attention and executive functioning. Additionally, the internalizing nature of ADHD symptoms in girls may lead clinicians and educators to overlook or attribute these behaviors to other causes, such as anxiety or depression.

Early intervention is crucial for girls with ADHD to address their unique needs and promote positive outcomes. By recognizing the signs and symptoms of ADHD in girls and seeking professional evaluation and diagnosis, parents can access the support and resources necessary to help their daughters succeed academically, socially, and emotionally. With early intervention, girls with ADHD can learn to harness their strengths, manage their challenges, and thrive in all areas of life.

Without early identification, girls with ADHD may be at risk for developing secondary complications, such as low self-esteem, academic underachievement, behavioral problems, and mental health disorders. These complications can have long-term consequences that impact girls' educational attainment, career opportunities, and quality of life.

Early intervention not only benefits girls with ADHD but also empowers their families and caregivers to better understand and support them. It helps parents and caregivers develop effective parenting strategies, advocate for their child's needs, and create supportive home environments that foster their daughter's growth and development.

Breaking Through Stereotypes

Societal expectations and gender norms play a significant role in shaping how ADHD manifests in girls. Girls are often expected to be quiet, compliant, and socially adept, making it easier for their symptoms to go under the radar. Recognizing the signs and symptoms of ADHD in girls is the first step towards providing them with the support and resources they need to thrive.

From struggles with organization and time management to difficulties in maintaining friendships and managing emotions, girls with ADHD face a myriad of challenges that may impact every aspect of their lives. Girls with ADHD often experience academic difficulties, including poor concentration, disorganization, and impulsivity, which can impact their learning and academic achievement.

Early diagnosis can help identify these challenges and provide targeted support, such as individualized education plans (IEPs), accommodations, and interventions to address specific learning needs. By addressing academic challenges early on, girls with ADHD can receive the support they need to succeed academically and reach their educational goals.

ADHD can also impact girls' social and emotional development, leading to difficulties in forming and maintaining friendships, regulating emotions, and coping with stress. Early intervention provides these girls with social skills training, cognitive-behavioral therapy (CBT), and other interventions to help them develop coping strategies, build resilience, and navigate social interactions more effectively.

By addressing social and emotional challenges early on, girls with ADHD can improve their self-esteem, confidence, and overall well-being. Whether you are a parent, caregiver, educator, or healthcare professional, we invite you to join us as we explore the world of ADHD through the lens of girls and discover the incredible potential that lies within each and every one of them.

As we embark on this journey of understanding ADHD in girls, let us challenge stereotypes, break down barriers, and advocate for greater awareness and support. By shining a light on the invisible struggles of girls with ADHD, we can create a more inclusive and compassionate society that empowers every individual to reach their full potential.

Let us embark on this transformative journey together, embracing leadership and empowering our girls to reach for the stars.

Welcome to the journey.

PART I: UNDERSTANDING ADHD IN GIRLS

In Part I of this book, we will delve into the complexities of ADHD as it pertains specifically to girls. By exploring the unique challenges, symptoms, and presentations of ADHD in girls, we aim to provide parents, caregivers, educators, and healthcare professionals with a deeper understanding of this often misunderstood condition.

Chapter 1: What is ADHD?

Attention-deficit hyperactivity disorder (ADHD) is a neurodevelopmental disorder that affects millions of individuals worldwide, yet its complexity and nuances continue to puzzle many. In this chapter, we aim to shed light on the fundamental aspects of ADHD, from its defining characteristics to its impact on daily life.

At its core, ADHD is characterized by a persistent pattern of inattention, hyperactivity, and impulsivity that interferes with functioning or development. Individuals with ADHD may struggle to focus, maintain attention, stay organized, or control impulses, leading to difficulties in academic, social, and occupational settings.

ADHD is further categorized into three main types: predominantly inattentive presentation, predominantly hyperactive-impulsive presentation, and combined presentation, which encompasses symptoms of both inattention and hyperactivity-impulsivity. Each subtype manifests differently, with some individuals exhibiting primarily inattentive symptoms, others displaying predominantly hyperactive-impulsive symptoms, and some experiencing a combination of both.

ADHD is believed to stem from complex interactions between genetic, environmental, and neurobiological factors. Neuroimaging studies have shown differences in brain structure and function among individuals with ADHD, particularly in regions associated with attention, impulse control, and executive function. Additionally, abnormalities in neurotransmitter systems, such as dopamine and norepinephrine, have been implicated in the etiology of ADHD.

ADHD is a multifaceted disorder characterized by difficulties in attention, hyperactivity, and impulsivity. While ADHD may present differently in girls compared to boys, it is essential to recognize and address the unique challenges faced by individuals of all genders.

Definition: Attention-deficit/hyperactivity disorder (ADHD) is a neurodevelopmental disorder characterized by a persistent pattern of inattention, hyperactivity, and impulsivity that interferes with functioning or development.

Now that we've seen the definition, let's read about the major symptoms of adhd.

Symptoms of ADHD

- **Inattention**: Individuals with ADHD may struggle to sustain attention, follow instructions, or complete tasks, leading to careless mistakes and difficulty organizing activities.
- **Hyperactivity**: Hyperactive behaviors may include excessive fidgeting, restlessness, or difficulty remaining seated, particularly in situations that require quiet or stillness.
- **Impulsivity**: Impulsive behaviors may manifest as acting without considering consequences, interrupting others, or blurting out answers before questions are completed.

Now that we've seen the symptoms, what about the types of ADHD available? ADHD is not a one-size-fits all. There are 3 distinct presentations that have been identified.

Types of ADHD

1) **Predominantly Inattentive Presentation:** This type of ADHD is characterized by primarily inattentive symptoms, such as difficulty focusing, forgetfulness, and disorganization, with minimal hyperactivity-impulsivity.

2) **Predominantly Hyperactive-Impulsive Presentation:** In contrast, this type of ADHD is characterized by predominantly hyperactive-impulsive symptoms, such as excessive fidgeting, impulsivity, and difficulty waiting for turn, with minimal inattention.

3) **Combined Presentation:** The combined presentation encompasses symptoms of both inattention and hyperactivity-impulsivity, making it the most common type of ADHD.

Subtypes and Variability

It's important to note that ADHD symptoms can vary widely among individuals, leading to variability in presentation and severity. Some individuals may exhibit predominantly inattentive symptoms, while others may display primarily hyperactive-impulsive symptoms. Additionally, the severity of symptoms can fluctuate over time and in different contexts, making ADHD a heterogeneous and complex disorder.

Given the variability in ADHD symptoms and presentations, it's crucial to conduct a comprehensive evaluation to accurately diagnose and tailor treatment for each individual. Treatment options for ADHD may include medication, behavioral therapy, educational interventions, and lifestyle modifications, depending on the specific needs and preferences of the individual.

Understanding the Neurobiology of ADHD

Attention-deficit hyperactivity disorder (ADHD) is not just a behavioral or psychological condition; it also has significant neurobiological underpinnings. Neuroimaging studies have revealed differences in brain structure and function among individuals with ADHD compared to those without the disorder. Specifically, areas of the brain involved in attention, impulse control, and executive function, such as the prefrontal cortex, basal ganglia, and cerebellum, show abnormalities in individuals with ADHD.

These differences may contribute to the difficulties in attention, hyperactivity, and impulsivity characteristic of the disorder. Dysregulation of neurotransmitter systems, particularly dopamine and norepinephrine, is thought to play a central role in the pathophysiology of ADHD. Both dopamine and norepinephrine are neurotransmitters involved in the regulation of attention, motivation, and reward processing.

Abnormalities in these neurotransmitter systems may lead to disruptions in neural circuits responsible for executive function and behavioral control, contributing to the core symptoms of ADHD. ADHD is highly heritable, with genetic factors estimated to account for around 70-80% of the variance in ADHD risk. Several genes implicated in dopamine and norepinephrine signaling pathways have been associated with an increased susceptibility to ADHD.

However, environmental factors, such as prenatal exposure to toxins, maternal smoking during pregnancy, and early life adversity, also play a role in the development of ADHD. Gene-environment interactions may further exacerbate the risk of ADHD and influence its severity and course. ADHD is a developmental disorder that often persists into adolescence and adulthood, albeit with varying degrees of symptom severity and impairment.

Longitudinal studies have shown that individuals with ADHD may experience delays in brain maturation and exhibit atypical developmental trajectories compared to neurotypical individuals. These developmental differences may contribute to ongoing difficulties in attention, impulse control, and academic achievement throughout the lifespan.

Implications for Treatment
Understanding the neurobiology of ADHD is essential for informing treatment approaches and interventions. Medications commonly used to treat ADHD, such as stimulants and non-stimulants, target dopamine and norepinephrine pathways to improve attention, focus, and impulse control. Behavioral interventions, such as cognitive-behavioral therapy (CBT) and psychoeducation, aim to teach individuals with ADHD coping strategies and organizational skills to manage their symptoms effectively.

ADHD is a complex neurodevelopmental disorder characterized by abnormalities in brain structure and function, dysregulation of neurotransmitter systems, and interactions between genetic and environmental factors. By unraveling the neurobiology of ADHD, we can gain insights into its underlying mechanisms and develop more targeted and effective treatments to support individuals affected by this disorder.

Gender Differences in ADHD Presentation

Societal expectations and gender norms play a significant role in shaping how ADHD symptoms are perceived and expressed in girls. Girls are often expected to be quiet, compliant, and socially adept, making it easier for their symptoms to go unnoticed or be dismissed. Instead of exhibiting overt hyperactivity and impulsivity, girls with ADHD may display more subtle symptoms, such as inattention, disorganization, and emotional dysregulation, which may be overlooked or attributed to other causes.

Girls with ADHD often exhibit symptoms that differ from those commonly associated with the disorder in boys. While boys with ADHD tend to display more externalizing behaviors such as hyperactivity and impulsivity, girls with ADHD often present with internalizing symptoms such as inattention, disorganization, and emotional dysregulation. As a result, their symptoms may be overlooked or misinterpreted, leading to delays in diagnosis.

While boys with ADHD tend to display more externalizing behaviors such as hyperactivity and impulsivity, girls with ADHD often present with internalizing symptoms such as inattention, disorganization, and emotional dysregulation.

The internalizing nature of ADHD symptoms in girls can make it difficult for parents, teachers, and healthcare professionals to recognize the disorder. Girls with ADHD may develop coping mechanisms to mask their symptoms, such as working harder to compensate for their difficulties or withdrawing from social situations to avoid embarrassment. These adaptive strategies may help girls blend in and appear "normal," making it less likely for them to receive a timely diagnosis.

Girls with ADHD often experience co-occurring conditions such as anxiety, depression, and eating disorders, which can complicate the diagnostic process. Symptoms of ADHD may be attributed to these comorbidities, leading to misdiagnosis or delayed diagnosis. Without proper recognition and treatment of ADHD, girls may continue to struggle academically, socially, and emotionally, impacting their overall well-being and quality of life.

Girls with ADHD are more likely to exhibit internalizing symptoms, such as daydreaming, forgetfulness, and difficulty staying organized, rather than the externalizing behaviors commonly associated with boys. Internalizing symptoms may include excessive worrying, perfectionism, and low self-esteem, which can mask underlying ADHD-related difficulties and lead to underdiagnosis or misdiagnosis.

Underdiagnosis and Misdiagnosis

Due to the differences in ADHD presentation between boys and girls, girls with ADHD are at a higher risk of being underdiagnosed or misdiagnosed. Girls with ADHD may be perceived as "quiet" or "well-behaved," leading to delays in recognizing their difficulties and seeking appropriate support and intervention. Additionally, symptoms of ADHD in girls may be misattributed to other conditions, such as anxiety, depression, or learning disabilities, further complicating the diagnostic process.

To address the underdiagnosis of ADHD in girls, it is essential to raise awareness and understanding of the gender differences in ADHD presentation. Educating parents, teachers, healthcare professionals, and the general public about the unique challenges faced by girls with ADHD can help improve early identification and intervention. Advocating for greater awareness and understanding can ensure that girls with ADHD receive the support and resources they need to thrive academically, socially, and emotionally.

Recognizing the gender differences in ADHD presentation is crucial for accurately identifying and supporting girls with ADHD. By understanding the societal expectations, internalizing behaviors, and challenges associated with diagnosing ADHD in girls, we can work towards creating a more inclusive and supportive environment for all individuals affected by this disorder.

Chapter 2: Recognizing ADHD in Girls

Recognizing attention deficit hyperactivity disorder (ADHD) in girls can be challenging due to the differences in how symptoms manifest compared to boys. In this chapter, we will explore the unique signs and symptoms of ADHD in girls and provide guidance on how to recognize and seek support for girls who may be struggling with the disorder.

Here are the subtle signs of inattention that may indicate that a girl has ADHD. There are so many subtleties that they may go unnoticed.

Subtle Signs of Inattention

→ **Daydreaming**: Girls with ADHD may spend a significant amount of time lost in thought, appearing distracted or unfocused during activities.
→ **Forgetfulness**: Forgetfulness and difficulty remembering instructions or completing tasks may be common in girls with ADHD.
→ **Disorganization**: Girls with ADHD may struggle with organization, often

misplacing belongings or having messy workspaces.

→ **Emotional Sensitivity:** Girls with ADHD may be more emotionally sensitive, experiencing mood swings, frustration, or tearfulness in response to stress or criticism.

→ **Low Self-Esteem**: Chronic underachievement and difficulties in school may contribute to low self-esteem and feelings of inadequacy in girls with ADHD.

→ **Perfectionism**: Some girls with ADHD may exhibit perfectionistic tendencies, striving for perfection to compensate for their underlying difficulties.

→ **Difficulty Maintaining Friendships:** Girls with ADHD may struggle to maintain friendships due to social awkwardness, impulsivity, or difficulty understanding social cues.

→ **Social Withdrawal**: Some girls with ADHD may withdraw from social situations to avoid embarrassment or rejection, leading to isolation and loneliness.

→ **Peer Rejection:** Girls with ADHD may be at risk of peer rejection due to differences in behavior or communication style, further exacerbating social difficulties.

→ **Poor Academic Performance:** Girls with ADHD may struggle academically due to difficulties with attention, organization, and time management.

→ **Inconsistent Work Habits**: Inconsistent work habits, such as procrastination or incomplete assignments, may be indicative of ADHD-related difficulties.

→ **Underachievement**: Despite their potential, girls with ADHD may underachieve academically, leading to frustration and disengagement from school.

A comprehensive evaluation, including clinical interviews, behavioral assessments, and rating scales, can help confirm the diagnosis and guide treatment planning. Early intervention, including medication, behavioral therapy, educational accommodations, and support services, can make a significant difference in improving outcomes and quality of life for girls with ADHD.

Recognizing ADHD in girls requires awareness of the subtle signs and symptoms, as well as an understanding of the unique challenges they may face. By identifying and addressing ADHD-related difficulties early on, we can help girls with ADHD thrive academically, socially, and emotionally, unlocking their full potential and supporting their success in all areas of life.

Common Signs and Symptoms of ADHD in Girls

Attention-deficit hyperactivity disorder (ADHD) can present differently in girls compared to boys, often leading to underdiagnosis or misdiagnosis. Recognizing the signs and symptoms of ADHD in girls is essential for early intervention and support. Below are a few typical indicators and manifestations to be mindful of:

1. Inattention
Difficulty Sustaining Focus: Girls with ADHD may struggle to stay focused on tasks, often becoming easily distracted or lost in thought.
Forgetfulness: Forgetfulness and absentmindedness are common, leading to missed appointments, lost items, and incomplete assignments.
Poor Organization: Girls with ADHD may have difficulty organizing tasks, materials, and

schedules, resulting in messy workspaces and difficulty managing time.

2. Hyperactivity

Restlessness: While hyperactivity may be less pronounced in girls with ADHD, they may still exhibit signs of restlessness, such as fidgeting or tapping their feet.

Excessive Talking: Girls with ADHD may talk excessively, blurting out answers or interrupting others in conversations.

Difficulty Staying Seated: They may have difficulty staying seated in situations where it is expected, such as during class or meals.

3. Impulsivity

Impulsive Decision-Making: Girls with ADHD may act impulsively without considering the consequences, leading to risky behaviors or impulsively making decisions.

Interrupting Others: They may have difficulty waiting their turn in conversations or games, frequently interrupting others or blurting out comments.

Difficulty Waiting: Waiting in line or waiting for their turn in activities may be challenging for girls with ADHD, leading to impatience and frustration.

4. Emotional Dysregulation

Mood Swings: Girls with ADHD may experience frequent mood swings, ranging from irritability and frustration to sadness or anxiety.

Sensitivity to Criticism: They may be more sensitive to criticism or rejection, reacting strongly to perceived slights or negative feedback.

Difficulty Coping with Stress: Coping with stress may be challenging for girls with ADHD, leading to feelings of overwhelm or avoidance of stressful situations.

5. Academic and Social Challenges

Underachievement: Academic underachievement is common among girls with ADHD, despite their potential, due to difficulties with attention, organization, and time management.

Social Withdrawal: Some girls with ADHD may withdraw from social activities or struggle to maintain friendships due to social awkwardness or difficulty understanding social cues.

Peer Rejection: Girls with ADHD may be at risk of peer rejection or bullying due to differences in behavior or communication style.

If you suspect that a girl may have ADHD based on these signs and symptoms, it is essential to seek support from healthcare professionals, educators, and mental health professionals. A comprehensive evaluation can help confirm the diagnosis and guide treatment planning, including medication, behavioral therapy, educational accommodations, and support services. Early intervention and support are key to helping girls with ADHD thrive academically, socially, and emotionally.

Gender-Specific Challenges

Girls with attention-deficit hyperactivity disorder (ADHD) often face unique challenges and may experience co-occurring conditions that require special attention and understanding. Girls with ADHD are more likely to go undiagnosed or misdiagnosed due to differences in symptom presentation compared to boys. Their symptoms may be overlooked or attributed to other conditions such as anxiety or depression, leading to delays in receiving appropriate support and intervention.

Girls with ADHD are more likely to exhibit internalizing symptoms such as inattention, emotional dysregulation, and social withdrawal, which may be less noticeable than the externalizing behaviors commonly seen in boys. This can make it challenging for parents, teachers, and healthcare professionals to recognize ADHD in girls.

Societal expectations and gender norms may influence how ADHD symptoms are perceived in girls. Girls are often expected to be quiet, compliant, and socially adept, making it easier for their symptoms to go unnoticed or be dismissed as typical girl behavior.

Co-occurring Conditions

Anxiety Disorders: Girls with ADHD are at an increased risk of developing anxiety disorders such as generalized anxiety disorder, social anxiety disorder, or separation anxiety disorder. The combination of ADHD and anxiety can exacerbate symptoms and impair functioning in various areas of life.

Depressive Disorders: Depression is common among girls with ADHD, particularly as they enter adolescence. Chronic underachievement, peer rejection, and low self-esteem associated with ADHD can contribute to the development of depressive symptoms.

Learning Disabilities: Girls with ADHD may also have co-occurring learning disabilities such as dyslexia or dyscalculia, which can further impact academic performance and exacerbate feelings of frustration and inadequacy.

Eating Disorders: There is evidence to suggest that girls with ADHD may be at a higher risk of developing eating disorders such as binge eating disorder or bulimia nervosa. Impulsivity, low self-esteem, and emotional dysregulation associated with ADHD may contribute to disordered eating behaviors.

Self-harm and Suicidal Behavior: Girls with ADHD are at an increased risk of engaging in self-harming behaviors or experiencing suicidal thoughts and behaviors, particularly in the presence of comorbid anxiety or depression.

Recognizing the gender-specific challenges and co-occurring conditions in girls with ADHD is essential for providing appropriate support and intervention. Early identification, comprehensive assessment, and targeted treatment can help address the unique needs of girls with ADHD and improve outcomes in academic, social, and emotional functioning. By understanding and addressing the complexities of ADHD in girls, we can better support their overall well-being and success.

Identifying ADHD Across Developmental Stages

Attention-deficit hyperactivity disorder (ADHD) can manifest differently at various stages of development, making it essential to recognize the signs and symptoms across different age groups.

Early Childhood (Preschool Age)

In preschool-aged children, hyperactive behavior may be more noticeable, including excessive fidgeting, running or climbing in inappropriate situations, and difficulty playing quietly. Impulsive behaviors such as interrupting others, grabbing toys from peers, or speaking out of turn may be evident. Signs of inattention, such as difficulty following instructions, forgetfulness, and frequently losing toys or other items, may also be observed.

Middle Childhood (Elementary School Age)

Inattention and impulsivity can impact academic performance, leading to difficulties completing assignments, staying organized, and paying attention in class. Girls with ADHD may struggle to maintain friendships, engage in cooperative play, or follow social rules, leading to peer rejection or social isolation.

Impulsivity and difficulty regulating emotions may contribute to behavioral problems such as aggression, defiance, or tantrums, particularly in structured settings like school or daycare.

Adolescence (Teenage Years)

Adolescent girls with ADHD may continue to struggle academically, experiencing difficulties with time management, planning, and organization, which can impact grades and academic achievement. Impulsivity and sensation-seeking tendencies may lead to risk-taking behaviors such as substance abuse, reckless driving, or unsafe sexual practices.

Adolescent girls with ADHD may experience heightened emotional reactivity, mood swings, and irritability, which can contribute to conflicts with peers, family members, and authority figures.

How to Identify ADHD

Observation and Screening: Parents, teachers, and healthcare professionals play a crucial role in observing and screening for ADHD symptoms across developmental stages. Screening tools such as behavior rating scales and checklists can help identify potential signs of ADHD. Go to www…. To take the test and see if you likely have adhd.

Comprehensive Assessment: A comprehensive assessment, including clinical interviews, behavioral observations, and standardized testing, is necessary to confirm the diagnosis of ADHD and rule out other potential causes of symptoms.

Collaboration and Communication: Collaboration between parents, educators, healthcare providers, and mental health professionals is essential for accurate diagnosis and treatment planning. Open communication and sharing of information about the child's behavior across different settings can provide valuable insights into ADHD symptoms.

By recognizing the signs and symptoms of ADHD across developmental stages and conducting thorough assessments, we can ensure early identification and intervention for children and adolescents with ADHD, leading to improved outcomes and quality of life.

Chapter 3: The Impact of ADHD on Girls

Attention-deficit hyperactivity disorder (ADHD) have significant effects on the lives of girls, impacting various aspects of their academic, social, and emotional well-being. Girls with ADHD may struggle academically due to difficulties with attention, organization and time management. This can lead to lower grades, academic underachievement, and feelings of frustration or inadequacy.

ADHD often co-occurs with learning disabilities such as dyslexia or dyscalculia, further complicating academic performance and exacerbating feelings of academic inadequacy. Impulsivity and difficulty regulating emotions may contribute to behavioral problems in school, such as defiance, disruption, or non-compliance with rules and instructions.

Girls with ADHD may struggle to maintain friendships or engage in social activities due to social awkwardness, difficulty understanding social cues, or emotional dysregulation. Differences in behavior or communication style may lead to peer rejection or bullying, further exacerbating feelings of social isolation and loneliness.

Impact of ADHD in Girls

Mood swings, irritability, and heightened emotional reactivity, intense emotions, difficulty coping with stress or frustration, chronic underachievement, peer rejection, social difficulties leading to low self-esteem and negative self-concept in girls.

Girls with ADHD may internalize feelings of inadequacy or failure, believing that they are not as competent or capable as their peers. Some girls with ADHD may experience imposter syndrome, feeling like they are constantly pretending to be someone they are not or that they do not deserve their achievements.

The impact of ADHD on girls extends beyond academic performance to affect their social relationships, emotional well-being, and self-esteem. By understanding the unique challenges faced by girls with ADHD and providing appropriate support and intervention, we can help them navigate their difficulties and thrive in all areas of life. Empowering girls with ADHD to recognize their strengths, seek support, and advocate for their needs is essential for promoting their overall health and happiness.

Academic Challenges and Learning Differences

Attention-deficit hyperactivity disorder (ADHD) can pose significant academic challenges for girls, often leading to learning differences and difficulties in educational settings. Here are the specific ways adhd affect the academic performance and learning differences for girls.

Academic Challenges

Inattention: Girls with ADHD may have difficulty sustaining attention and focusing on tasks, leading to missed instructions, incomplete assignments, and poor academic performance.

Organization: Executive function deficits associated with ADHD can manifest as disorganization, forgetfulness, and difficulty managing time and materials, making it challenging to stay on top of schoolwork and assignments.

Time Management: Girls with ADHD may struggle with time management skills, leading to procrastination, rushing through assignments, and difficulty meeting deadlines.

Reading and Writing Skills: Some girls with ADHD may experience difficulties with reading comprehension, writing fluency, and spelling, which can impact their ability to understand and express themselves effectively in written assignments.

Mathematics: Problems with attention, working memory, and processing speed may contribute to difficulties with mathematical concepts, problem-solving, and arithmetic calculations.

Learning Differences

Processing Speed: Girls with ADHD may exhibit slower processing speed, affecting their ability to quickly absorb and respond to information in academic tasks and assessments.

Working Memory: Deficits in working memory can impact a girl's ability to hold and manipulate information in her mind, making it challenging to follow multi-step instructions or remember important details.

Executive Functioning: Executive function deficits, including difficulties with planning, organization, and self-regulation, can hinder a girl's ability to manage academic tasks independently and efficiently.

Attentional Control: Impaired attentional control can lead to distractibility, impulsivity, and difficulty filtering out irrelevant information in the classroom, affecting learning and retention of new material.

Visual-Spatial Skills: Some girls with ADHD may struggle with visual-spatial skills, making it difficult to interpret diagrams, maps, or graphs and understand spatial relationships in geometry or science.

Even though adhd adversely affects girls, all hope is not lost. There are some interventions that can help with specifically academic challenges.

Addressing Academic Challenges

Individualized Education Plans (IEPs) or 504 Plans: Girls with ADHD may benefit from accommodations and support outlined in an IEP or 504 Plan, such as extra time during tests and exams, special seating arrangements, or tools for organization.

Multimodal Instruction: Providing instruction through multiple modalities, such as visual aids, hands-on activities, and auditory cues, can help accommodate different learning styles and support girls with ADHD.

Structured Routines and Schedules: Establishing structured routines and schedules can help girls with ADHD manage their time, stay organized, and prioritize tasks effectively.

Positive Reinforcement: Encouraging and reinforcing positive behaviors and achievements can boost motivation and self-esteem in girls with ADHD, fostering a positive attitude towards learning.

Collaboration with Teachers and Support Staff: Open communication and collaboration between parents, teachers, and support staff are essential for identifying and addressing the academic needs of girls with ADHD effectively.

By recognizing the academic challenges and learning differences faced by girls with ADHD and implementing appropriate strategies and supports, we can help them overcome obstacles and achieve academic success. Empowering girls with ADHD to advocate for their needs, build resilience, and cultivate their strengths is key to promoting their overall educational attainment and well-being.

Social and Emotional Implications

Attention-deficit hyperactivity disorder (ADHD) can have profound effects on the social and emotional well-being of girls, impacting their relationships, self-esteem, and overall quality of life.

Difficulty Maintaining Friendships: Girls with ADHD may struggle to establish and maintain friendships due to social awkwardness, impulsivity, and difficulty understanding social cues. They may have trouble following social rules or taking turns in conversations and activities.

Peer Rejection: Differences in behavior or communication style may lead to peer rejection or exclusion, causing girls with ADHD to feel isolated and lonely. Repeated experiences of peer rejection can contribute to feelings of inadequacy and low self-esteem.

Social Anxiety: Some girls with ADHD may experience social anxiety or fear of judgment from peers, leading to avoidance of social situations or withdrawal from social activities. Social anxiety can further exacerbate social difficulties and impair social functioning.

Mood Swings: Girls with ADHD may experience frequent and intense mood swings, ranging from irritability and frustration to sadness or anxiety. These mood fluctuations can be triggered by external stressors or internal frustrations related to ADHD-related difficulties.

Emotional Sensitivity: Girls with ADHD may be more emotionally sensitive, reacting strongly to criticism, rejection, or perceived failures. They may have difficulty regulating their emotions and expressing themselves in socially appropriate ways.

Impulsivity and Reactivity: Impulsivity associated with ADHD can lead to impulsive outbursts or emotional reactions, such as sudden anger or frustration. Girls with ADHD may struggle to control their impulses and may lash out verbally or physically in response to perceived threats or frustrations.

Low Self-Esteem: Chronic underachievement, peer rejection, and social difficulties associated with ADHD can contribute to low self-esteem and negative self-concept in girls. They may internalize feelings of inadequacy or failure, believing that they are not as competent or capable as their peers.

Perfectionism: Some girls with ADHD may develop perfectionistic tendencies as a coping mechanism to compensate for their underlying difficulties. They may strive for perfection to prove their worth or to avoid criticism and rejection from others.

Imposter Syndrome: Imposter syndrome, characterized by feelings of self-doubt and fear of being exposed as a fraud, may be common among girls with ADHD. They may feel like they are constantly pretending to be someone they are not or that they do not deserve their achievements.

The social and emotional implications of ADHD in girls are profound and can significantly impact their well-being and quality of life. By recognizing the unique social and emotional challenges faced by girls with ADHD and providing appropriate support and intervention, we can help them navigate their difficulties and thrive in all areas of life. Empowering girls with ADHD to develop coping skills, build resilience, and cultivate supportive relationships is essential for promoting their overall social and emotional health.

Practical Coping Mechanisms and Adaptive Strategies

Girls with attention-deficit/hyperactivity disorder (ADHD) often face unique challenges in managing their symptoms and navigating daily life. However, there are several coping mechanisms and adaptive strategies that can help girls with ADHD better manage their symptoms and thrive in various settings. In this section, we will explore some effective coping mechanisms and adaptive strategies for girls with ADHD.

1. Time Management Techniques

Use of Visual Aids: Girls with ADHD can benefit from using visual aids such as planners, calendars, or digital apps to help them organize their tasks, appointments, and deadlines.

Color-coded Calendars: Use different colors to categorize tasks and appointments (e.g., blue for work/school, red for personal appointments, green for social events).

Time-blocking: Assign specific time slots for different activities or tasks throughout the day, and visually block off these periods on a calendar or planner.

Chunking: Chunking involves dividing large tasks into smaller, more manageable steps. Instead of tackling a daunting task like "cleaning the house" all at once, it is more effective to break it down into specific tasks such as "vacuuming the living room" or "washing dishes." This approach allows for better organization and makes the overall task seem less overwhelming.

Checklists: Create checklists or to-do lists for each day or week, outlining the specific steps needed to complete various tasks.

Pomodoro Technique: The Pomodoro Technique suggests setting a timer for 25 minutes of concentrated work, followed by a 5-minute break. Repeat this cycle (known as a "Pomodoro") several times, with longer breaks after every 4 cycles.

Use alarms: Set alarms or reminders on your phone or computer to prompt you to start or switch tasks at designated times.

ABC prioritization: Assign tasks to categories (A, B, C) based on their urgency and importance. Focus on completing high-priority tasks (A) before moving on to less urgent ones (B, C).

Eat the frog: Start your day by tackling the most challenging or important task first, rather than procrastinating and leaving it for later.

Create a dedicated workspace: Designate a specific area for work or study, free from distractions like TV, social media, or clutter.

Use noise-canceling headphones: Block out distractions by listening to white noise or calming music with noise-canceling headphones.

Task management apps: Use apps like Todoist, Trello, or Asana to organize tasks, set deadlines, and track progress.

Digital calendars: Sync your calendar across devices and set up reminders for appointments, deadlines, and important events.

Estimate task duration: Develop a better sense of how long tasks take to complete by estimating their duration before starting.

Track time spent: Use a timer or time-tracking app to monitor how much time you spend on different activities throughout the day, helping you become more aware of where your time goes.

Buffer time: Allow extra time between tasks or appointments to account for unexpected delays or transitions. This helps prevent feeling rushed or overwhelmed by tight schedules.

Remember that everyone's ADHD experience is unique, so it may take some trial and error to find the time management techniques that work best for you. Experiment with different strategies, be patient with yourself, and celebrate your successes along the way!

2. Organization Strategies

Establishing Routines: Creating structured routines and schedules can help girls with ADHD stay organized and manage their time more effectively. Consistent routines can also reduce anxiety and improve predictability. Develop consistent daily routines and rituals for activities such as waking up, meal times, work/study periods, and bedtime.

Utilizing Organizational Tools: Girls can use organizational tools such as color-coded folders, bins, or labels to keep track of their belongings and maintain an orderly environment.. For example, use different colored folders or labels to categorize documents or tasks based on priority or category.

Designate specific storage areas: Assign a designated place for commonly used items such as keys, wallet, or phone. Use baskets, bins, or shelves to keep items organized and easily accessible.

Clear workspace: Keep your work or study area clutter-free by regularly decluttering and organizing. Remove unnecessary items from your desk or workspace to minimize distractions.

Utilize Technology for Organization: Digital calendars and planners: Use digital calendars, planners, or task management apps to schedule appointments, set reminders, and track deadlines. Ensure convenient access to your calendar by synchronizing it across all your devices.

Note-taking apps: Use note-taking apps like Evernote or OneNote to capture ideas, reminders, and important information in one centralized location.

Establish Organization Habits: Daily organization routines: Incorporate daily organization habits into your routine, such as tidying up your workspace before starting work or setting aside time each day to sort through mail or paperwork.

Regular decluttering: Schedule regular decluttering sessions to purge unnecessary items and keep your living and work spaces organized.

Professional organizers: Consider hiring a professional organizer who specializes in working with individuals with ADHD. They can provide personalized strategies and support to help you create and maintain an organized environment.

Accountability partners: Partner with a friend, family member, or coach who can provide accountability and support as you work on improving your organization skills.

3. Self-Regulation Techniques

Mindfulness and Relaxation Exercises: Practicing mindfulness techniques or relaxation exercises can help girls with ADHD reduce stress, increase focus, improve emotional regulation, reduce impulsivity, and enhance self-awareness.

Deep Breathing or Progressive Muscle Relaxation: Encouraging girls to engage in deep breathing exercises or progressive muscle relaxation can help them calm their minds and bodies during times of stress or emotional dysregulation. Take a deep breath through your nostrils, retain it for a brief period, and then exhale gradually through your mouth.

Regular exercise: Engage in regular physical activity such as walking, jogging, swimming, or yoga to help regulate energy levels and improve mood. Exercise releases endorphins, which can boost mood and reduce symptoms of ADHD.

Fidget tools: Use fidget tools or toys (e.g., stress balls, fidget spinners) during sedentary activities to help channel excess energy and improve focus.

Scheduled breaks: Take regular breaks during tasks or activities to prevent burnout and maintain focus. Set a timer or schedule specific break times to ensure you step away from work or study periodically.

Restorative activities: Engage in restorative activities during breaks, such as listening to calming music, taking a short walk, or practicing relaxation techniques.

Journaling: Keep a journal to track thoughts, feelings, and behaviors throughout the day. Reflect on patterns or triggers for ADHD symptoms and identify strategies that help manage symptoms effectively.

Check-ins: Conduct regular check-ins with yourself to assess your current state of mind and energy levels. Adjust your activities or environment as needed to maintain optimal focus and productivity.

Time-blocking: Implement time-blocking to allocate dedicated time slots for various tasks or activities throughout the day. Use a timer or digital calendar to track time spent on each task and help maintain focus and productivity.

Prioritization: Prioritize tasks based on urgency and importance, focusing on completing high-priority tasks first. Divide extensive tasks into smaller, more feasible steps to avoid becoming overwhelmed.

Cognitive restructuring: Challenge negative thoughts and beliefs that may contribute to feelings of overwhelm or self-doubt. Substitute pessimistic thoughts with more practical and optimistic alternatives.

Problem-solving: Use problem-solving techniques to address challenges or obstacles as they arise. Break down problems into smaller components, brainstorm potential solutions, and implement a plan of action.

Seek support: Seek emotional support and encouragement from friends, family, or support groups. Share your experiences and challenges with others who understand and can offer empathy and understanding.

Remember that self-regulation techniques may need to be adapted and personalized to suit your individual preferences and needs. Experiment with different strategies, be patient with yourself, and celebrate your progress along the way!

4. Social Skills Training

Role-Playing Scenarios: Role-playing social scenarios with girls can help them practice appropriate social behaviors, such as taking turns, active listening, or initiating conversations.

Using Social Scripts: Providing girls with ADHD with social scripts or prompts for common social situations can help them navigate social interactions more confidently and effectively.

Body language: Pay attention to your body language, such as posture, facial expressions, and gestures, to convey interest and openness in social interactions. Practice using appropriate facial expressions to convey emotions and intentions in social interactions.

Ask clarifying questions: Ask questions to clarify any points that are unclear or to show interest in the conversation. Repeat back what the speaker has said in your own words to ensure understanding and demonstrate active listening.

Maintain eye contact: Practice making and maintaining eye contact with the speaker to demonstrate attentiveness and engagement.

Personal space: Respect others' personal space and boundaries by maintaining an appropriate distance during conversations. Take turns speaking in conversations, allowing others to share their thoughts and opinions without interruption.

Initiating conversations: Practice initiating conversations with others by asking open-ended questions or making observations about shared interests or experiences.

Topic maintenance: Stay on topic during conversations and avoid going off on tangents. Practice transitioning between topics smoothly and naturally.

Put yourself in others' shoes: Practice empathy by trying to understand others' perspectives, feelings, and experiences.

Active listening: Listen attentively to others' concerns and validate their feelings by acknowledging and empathizing with their experiences.

Expressing opinions: Practice expressing your opinions, thoughts, and feelings assertively and respectfully in social situations.

Negotiation skills: Develop negotiation skills to resolve conflicts or disagreements in a constructive and collaborative manner.

Setting boundaries: Learn to set and communicate clear boundaries with others to protect your own needs and well-being in social interactions.

Identify social cues: Practice recognizing and interpreting social cues, such as facial expressions, tone of voice, and body language, to better understand social situations.

Generate solutions: Brainstorm potential solutions to social problems or challenges, considering the perspectives and needs of all parties involved.

Evaluate outcomes: Reflect on the outcomes of social interactions and problem-solving efforts, identifying strategies that were effective and areas for improvement.

Real-life practice: Seek out opportunities to practice social skills in real-life settings, such as joining social groups, volunteering, or participating in social activities.

5. Study Strategies

Creating a Distraction-Free Environment: Girls with ADHD can benefit from studying in a quiet, clutter-free environment with minimal distractions, free from distractions such as noise, clutter, or electronic devices to help them stay focused and attentive.

Implementing Active Learning Techniques: Encouraging girls to use active learning techniques such as summarizing information, teaching material to someone else, or creating visual aids can enhance comprehension and retention of information.

Use noise-canceling headphones: Block out distractions by listening to calming music or white noise with noise-canceling headphones.

Limit access to distractions: Turn off notifications on your phone, close unnecessary browser tabs, and use website blockers if needed to minimize distractions during study sessions.

Set time limits: Use a timer to break study sessions into shorter intervals (e.g., 25 minutes of focused study followed by a 5-minute break) to maintain focus and productivity.

Mind maps: Create visual representations of concepts or ideas using mind maps or diagrams to help organize information and make connections between different concepts.

Color-coded notes: Use different colors to highlight key points, concepts, or categories in your notes. This can help improve memory retention and make studying more engaging.

Digital organizers: Use digital tools such as calendars, task lists, or note-taking apps to organize study materials, set reminders, and track progress on assignments and deadlines.

Practice retrieval: Use active recall techniques such as self-quizzing or flashcards to test your knowledge and reinforce learning.

Teach the material: Pretend to teach the material to someone else or explain concepts out loud in your own words to reinforce understanding and retention.

Apply concepts: Apply what you've learned to real-life examples of problem-solving scenarios to deepen your understanding and practical application of the material.

Use tactile methods: Engage multiple senses by using tactile learning methods such as writing out notes by hand, using manipulatives, or acting out concepts to reinforce learning.

Listen to recordings: Record lectures or readings and listen to them while engaging in other activities (e.g., walking, exercising) to reinforce auditory learning.

Prioritize tasks: Identify high-priority tasks and allocate your study time accordingly. Focus on completing tasks that are due soon or require immediate attention.

Use a planner: Use a planner or calendar to schedule study sessions, assignments, and exams, and stick to your study schedule as much as possible.

Scheduled breaks: Take regular breaks during study sessions to prevent burnout and maintain focus. Use breaks to rest, recharge, and engage in self-care activities.

Exercise and relaxation: Incorporate regular exercise, relaxation techniques, and stress management strategies into your routine to support overall well-being and enhance focus and productivity.

6. Seeking Support and Advocacy

Building a Support Network: Encouraging girls with ADHD to seek support from family, friends, teachers, and mental health professionals can provide them with the encouragement, validation, and guidance they need to navigate their challenges.

Research ADHD: Take the time to learn about ADHD, including its symptoms, challenges, and treatment options. Knowledge empowers you to better understand your own needs and advocate effectively for yourself.

Educate others: Share accurate information about ADHD with friends, family members, teachers, employers, and healthcare professionals to raise awareness and reduce stigma surrounding the condition.

Join support groups: Seek out local or online support groups for individuals with ADHD to connect with others who understand your experiences and can offer empathy, advice, and encouragement.

Connect with peers: Build supportive relationships with peers who have ADHD or similar challenges. They can provide understanding, validation, and practical tips for coping with everyday struggles.

Be open and honest: Communicate openly with teachers, employers, healthcare providers, and others about your ADHD diagnosis and how it impacts your daily life. Advocate for the accommodations and support you need to succeed.

Ask for help when needed: Don't hesitate to ask for help or clarification when you need it. Whether it's seeking academic accommodations, requesting workplace adjustments, or accessing mental health services, advocating for yourself is essential.

Find a healthcare provider: Work with a knowledgeable healthcare provider, such as a psychiatrist, psychologist, or therapist, who specializes in ADHD diagnosis and treatment. They can provide guidance, support, and evidence-based interventions tailored to your unique needs.

Consider therapy: Therapy, such as cognitive-behavioral therapy (CBT) or coaching, can help you develop coping skills, improve time management, and address emotional challenges related to ADHD.

Explore academic accommodations: If you're a student, work with your school's disability services office to access accommodations such as extended time on exams, note-taking assistance, or preferential seating.

Access workplace accommodations: If you're employed, discuss potential accommodations with your employer, such as flexible work hours, task prioritization assistance, or noise-reducing headphones.

Participate in advocacy efforts: Get involved in ADHD advocacy organizations and initiatives that work to raise awareness, promote research, and advocate for policy changes to support individuals with ADHD.

Share your story: Share your personal experiences with ADHD through writing, speaking engagements, social media, or community events to help educate others and reduce stigma.

Know your rights: Familiarize yourself with your legal rights and protections under laws such as the Americans with Disabilities Act (ADA) and the Individuals with Disabilities Education Act (IDEA).

Speak up for yourself: Be assertive in expressing your needs, preferences, and boundaries in various settings, whether it's in the classroom, workplace, healthcare setting, or social interactions.

By implementing these coping mechanisms and adaptive strategies, girls with ADHD can develop the skills and resources they need to manage their symptoms effectively and achieve success in various aspects of their lives. It is essential to provide girls with ADHD with the support, encouragement, and resources they need to thrive academically, socially, and emotionally. With the right tools and support, girls with ADHD can reach their full potential and lead fulfilling and successful lives.

Understanding and Parenting Your Girl Child with ADHD

PART II: PARENTING STRATEGIES FOR GIRLS WITH ADHD

Parenting a child with attention-deficit hyperactivity disorder (ADHD) presents unique challenges, particularly when it comes to supporting girls with ADHD who may exhibit different symptom patterns and coping mechanisms compared to boys. In this section, we will explore effective parenting strategies tailored to the needs of girls with ADHD, aimed at promoting their academic, social, and emotional well-being.

Chapter 4: Navigating Diagnosis and Treatment

Navigating the diagnosis and treatment process for girls with attention-deficit hyperactivity disorder (ADHD) requires careful consideration and proactive involvement from parents, caregivers, educators, and healthcare professionals.

The first step is seeking a qualified mental health professional, ideally someone experienced in diagnosing ADHD. This could be a psychiatrist, psychologist, or a licensed therapist specializing in ADHD. The evaluation process typically involves:

- In-depth interviews: Discussing your experiences, challenges, and family history.
- Symptom checklists: Standardized tools to assess the presence and severity of ADHD symptoms.
- Psychological testing (optional): In some cases, additional testing may be recommended to rule out other conditions with similar symptoms.

But before you go, you should be aware of the potential signs and symptoms of ADHD in girls, which may include inattention, distractibility, impulsivity, hyperactivity, emotional dysregulation, and difficulty with organization and time management. Observe your daughter's behavior across different settings and situations, including at home, school, and social settings, to identify any consistent patterns of behavior that may indicate ADHD.

Then schedule an appointment with your daughter's primary care physician or pediatrician to discuss your concerns about her behavior and request a referral for further evaluation by a specialist. Seek a referral to a qualified specialist, such as a child psychiatrist, pediatric neurologist, or clinical psychologist, with expertise in assessing and diagnosing ADHD in girls.

Provide a comprehensive medical history, including information about your daughter's developmental milestones, academic performance, social interactions, and any family history of ADHD or other mental health conditions. She may undergo a thorough behavioral assessment, which may involve standardized questionnaires, interviews, and behavioral observations, to assess your daughter's ADHD symptoms and functional impairment.

Ensure that the evaluation includes screening for common co-occurring conditions that may accompany ADHD, such as learning disabilities, anxiety disorders, depression, or autism spectrum disorder. Seek a comprehensive assessment that considers the full range of your daughter's strengths, challenges, and individual needs to inform diagnosis and treatment planning effectively.

Maintain open communication with the evaluating professionals, asking questions, expressing concerns, and advocating for your daughter's needs throughout the evaluation process. Seek clear and comprehensive feedback from the evaluating professionals regarding the results of the evaluation, including the diagnosis of ADHD, any co-occurring conditions, and recommended treatment options.

Work with the evaluating professionals to develop an individualized treatment plan tailored to your daughter's specific needs, which may include behavioral interventions, academic accommodations, medication management, and therapeutic support.

By following the steps outlined above and collaborating with qualified healthcare professionals, you as a parent can ensure an accurate diagnosis and effective treatment planning for their daughters with ADHD, enabling individuals to achieve their maximum potential and live satisfying lives.

Exploring Treatment Options: Medication, Therapy, and Other Approaches

Finding the most effective treatment approach for girls with attention-deficit hyperactivity disorder (ADHD) involves considering a range of options, including medication, therapy, and alternative approaches.

1. Medication: The first is stimulant medications such as methylphenidate (e.g., Ritalin, Concerta) and amphetamine (e.g., Adderall, Vyvanse) are commonly prescribed to manage ADHD symptoms in girls. These medications help improve attention, focus, and impulse control by increasing the levels of neurotransmitters in the brain.

The second is non-stimulant medications like atomoxetine (Strattera) and guanfacine (Intuniv) which may be prescribed as alternatives or adjuncts to stimulant medications, particularly for girls who do not respond well to stimulants or have co-occurring conditions.

2. Therapy: Behavioral therapy approaches such as cognitive-behavioral therapy (CBT) and behavioral parent training can help girls with ADHD develop coping skills, improve self-regulation, and manage challenging behaviors. These therapies focus on teaching practical strategies for managing ADHD symptoms in daily life.

Social skills training programs can help girls with ADHD improve their social competence, communication skills, and peer interactions. These programs teach essential social skills such as listening, taking turns, and resolving conflicts effectively.

Family therapy can be beneficial for girls with ADHD and their families, providing a supportive environment to address family dynamics, communication patterns, and parenting strategies. Family therapy can help improve parent-child relationships and enhance family functioning.

3. Alternative Approaches: Some parents explore dietary modifications, such as eliminating artificial additives, reducing sugar intake, or incorporating omega-3 fatty acids, to manage ADHD symptoms in girls. While research on the effectiveness of dietary interventions for ADHD is mixed, some girls may benefit from dietary changes.

Mindfulness practices, relaxation exercises, and yoga can help girls with ADHD reduce stress, improve self-awareness, and enhance emotional regulation. These practices promote mindfulness, self-reflection, and inner calmness.

Regular physical activity and exercise can have positive effects on ADHD symptoms, including improved attention, mood, and self-esteem. Encouraging girls with ADHD to engage in sports, outdoor activities, or structured exercise programs can help manage their symptoms.

4. Comprehensive Treatment Approach:
Work with healthcare professionals to develop
an individualized treatment plan that addresses
your daughter's specific needs, preferences,
and goals. A comprehensive approach may
involve a combination of medication, therapy,
and alternative approaches tailored to her
unique challenges.

Exploring treatment options for girls with ADHD
involves considering a range of approaches,
including medication, therapy, and alternative
interventions. By tailoring treatment to your
daughter's individual needs and preferences,
you can help her manage her ADHD symptoms
effectively and thrive in all areas of her life.

Advocating for Your Child's Needs in School and Community Settings

Advocating for your child with attention-deficit
hyperactivity disorder (ADHD) in school and
community settings is essential to ensure they
receive the support and accommodations
necessary to thrive academically, socially, and
emotionally. To do effectively, you need to:

❖ Familiarize yourself with your child's rights under relevant laws and regulations, such as the Individuals with Disabilities Education Act (IDEA), Section 504 of the Rehabilitation Act, and the Americans with Disabilities Act (ADA). Understand the eligibility criteria for special education services and accommodations for students with ADHD.

❖ Review the policies and procedures of your child's school regarding special education services, accommodations, and disciplinary practices. Understand the process for requesting evaluations, developing individualized education plans (IEPs), or implementing 504 plans.

❖ Develop positive relationships with your child's teachers, administrators, and support staff by fostering open communication and collaboration. Keep them informed about your child's diagnosis, strengths, challenges, and treatment plan.

- ❖ Attend meetings with school personnel, such as IEP meetings or parent-teacher conferences, to discuss your child's progress, review educational goals, and advocate for necessary accommodations or modifications.

- ❖ If you suspect that your child may have ADHD or other learning difficulties, request a comprehensive evaluation by the school's multidisciplinary team to assess their educational needs and eligibility for special education services.

- ❖ Monitor Progress: Regularly monitor your child's academic progress, social interactions, and emotional well-being to identify any areas of concern or areas where additional support may be needed.

- ❖ Follow-Up Meetings: Schedule follow-up meetings with school personnel to review your child's IEP or 504 plan, discuss their progress towards educational goals, and make any necessary adjustments to accommodations or services.

- ❖ Connecting with Support Groups: Seek out support groups or advocacy organizations for parents of children with ADHD to connect with other families facing similar challenges, share resources and strategies, and advocate collectively for improved services and supports.

- ❖ Utilizing Community Resources: Explore community resources and programs that may provide additional support and services for children with ADHD, such as tutoring programs, behavioral therapy services, or recreational activities tailored to their interests.

- ❖ Encourage Self-Advocacy: Teach your child self-advocacy skills, such as expressing their needs, asking for help when needed, and advocating for themselves in school and community settings. Help them understand their rights and responsibilities as a student with ADHD.

- ❖ Promote Self-Esteem: Foster a sense of self-esteem and confidence in your child by emphasizing their strengths, celebrating their achievements, and providing positive reinforcement for their efforts.

By understanding your child's rights, building collaborative relationships with school personnel, and actively advocating for their needs, you can help create an inclusive and supportive environment that enables your child to reach their full potential despite the challenges of ADHD. Remember to prioritize communication, monitor progress, seek community support, and empower your child to become their own advocate in navigating their educational journey.

Chapter 5: Building a Supportive Environment

Creating a supportive environment is crucial for girls with attention-deficit hyperactivity disorder (ADHD) to thrive academically, socially, and emotionally. Here are the ways to build a supportive environment for your daughter and the girls around you.

Educate family members, including siblings, parents, grandparents, and extended family, about ADHD and its impact on girls. Foster understanding and acceptance of your daughter's unique needs, strengths, and challenges.Use positive, strengths-based language when discussing ADHD with your daughter and others. Avoid stigmatizing or negative language that may contribute to feelings of shame or inadequacy.

Create structured daily routines and schedules for your daughter, including set times for meals, homework, bedtime, and extracurricular activities. Consistent routines provide predictability and stability, which can help girls with ADHD manage their symptoms more effectively. Use visual aids such as calendars, checklists, and timers to help your daughter understand and follow routines. Visual support can enhance organization, time management, and task completion for girls with ADHD.

Clearly communicate expectations for behavior, chores, and academic tasks to your daughter, breaking tasks down into manageable steps. Provide specific, positive feedback and praise for her efforts and accomplishments. Implement reinforcement systems such as token economies, behavior charts, or reward systems to motivate your daughter and reinforce positive behaviors. Consistent reinforcement can help girls with ADHD stay motivated and engaged.

Foster open, honest communication with your daughter, encouraging her to express her thoughts, feelings, and concerns. Listen actively and validate her experiences, showing empathy and understanding. Teach your daughter problem-solving skills and strategies for overcoming challenges. Encourage her to brainstorm solutions, evaluate options, and make decisions independently.

Offer emotional support and validation to your daughter, acknowledging the challenges she faces and expressing confidence in her abilities to overcome them. Be a source of comfort, reassurance, and encouragement during difficult times. Teach your daughter coping strategies such as deep breathing exercises, mindfulness techniques, or sensory self-regulation strategies to help her manage stress, anxiety, and emotional dysregulation.

Collaborate with your daughter's teachers, school counselors, and administrators to develop a supportive learning environment that meets her needs. Advocate for appropriate accommodations, modifications, and support services in the classroom. Explore community resources and support services available to girls with ADHD and their families, such as support groups, counseling services, recreational programs, and educational workshops.

Building a supportive environment for girls with ADHD requires understanding, patience, and proactive intervention. By establishing structured routines, setting clear expectations, fostering effective communication, providing emotional support, and collaborating with schools and communities, you can create an environment that empowers your daughter to thrive despite the challenges of ADHD.

Creating Structure and Routine at Home

Establishing structure and routine at home is essential for girls with attention-deficit hyperactivity disorder (ADHD) to thrive and manage their symptoms effectively. Here are some practical strategies for creating a supportive and organized environment that promotes success and well-being for girls with ADHD.

1. **Establish Consistent Daily Routines:** Establish consistent wake-up and bedtime routines for your daughter to ensure she gets an adequate amount of sleep each night. Consistent sleep schedules can help regulate her mood, attention, and behavior. Develop structured daily schedules that outline specific times for activities such as meals, homework, chores, playtime, and relaxation. Display the schedules visually using calendars or whiteboards to provide visual cues and reminders.

2. **Break Tasks into Manageable Steps:**
Break down tasks and responsibilities into
smaller, more manageable steps to prevent
overwhelm and facilitate task completion.
Create checklists or task lists for your daughter
to follow, highlighting each step in the process.
Clearly communicate instructions and
expectations for tasks and chores, using
simple language and concrete examples. Avoid
vague or open-ended instructions that may be
confusing for girls with ADHD.

3. **Utilize Visual Supports and Reminders:**
Use visual schedules or picture charts to help
your daughter understand and follow daily
routines and transitions. Include visual cues for
each activity or task to provide guidance and
structure. Set up reminder systems such as
alarms, timers, or smartphone apps to help
your daughter stay on track with her schedule
and responsibilities. Use auditory and visual
reminders to prompt her to start or complete
tasks.

4. **Implement Consistent Rules and
Expectations:** Develop clear and consistent
household rules and expectations for behavior,
chores, screen time, and social interactions.
Review the rules regularly with your daughter

and enforce them consistently. Reinforce positive behaviors and accomplishments with praise, rewards, or privileges to motivate your daughter and reinforce desired behaviors. Focus on acknowledging her efforts and progress, rather than just outcomes.

5. **Create Organized Study Spaces:** Set up designated study areas in quiet, clutter-free environments where your daughter can focus and concentrate on her schoolwork. Remove distractions such as electronics or noisy activities from these spaces. Equip study areas with organizational tools such as desks, drawers, shelving units, and school supplies to help your daughter stay organized and keep track of her materials.

6. **Promote Self-Care and Relaxation:** Encourage your daughter to take regular breaks during study sessions or other tasks to prevent fatigue and maintain focus. Incorporate short breaks for physical activity, relaxation, or mindfulness exercises. Model healthy self-care practices such as regular exercise, balanced nutrition, adequate sleep, and stress management techniques for your daughter to emulate. Prioritize self-care as a family value.

Creating structure and routine at home is essential for girls with ADHD to feel organized, supported, and successful in managing their symptoms and daily responsibilities.

Setting Clear Expectations and Boundaries

Setting clear expectations and boundaries is crucial for girls with attention-deficit hyperactivity disorder (ADHD) to understand what is expected of them and to navigate their daily routines successfully. Let's explore practical strategies for establishing clear expectations and boundaries to promote positive behavior and support your daughter's development.

When setting expectations and boundaries, use simple and straightforward language that is easy for your daughter to understand. Avoid using vague or ambiguous terms that may confuse her. Clearly outline your expectations for behavior, chores, academic tasks, and social interactions. Provide specific examples and explanations to illustrate what is expected in different situations.

Identify the most important rules and boundaries that are essential for maintaining a safe, orderly, and harmonious home environment. Focus on rules that address safety, respect, responsibility, and cooperation. Enforce rules consistently and fairly, ensuring that consequences for breaking rules are predictable and proportionate to the behavior. Avoid making exceptions or changing consequences on a whim.

Assign age-appropriate chores and responsibilities to your daughter based on her abilities and developmental level. Break tasks down into manageable steps and provide guidance and support as needed. Incorporate chores and responsibilities into daily routines and schedules to ensure they become habitual and predictable. Use visual reminders and checklists to help your daughter remember her tasks.

Create a safe and supportive environment where your daughter feels comfortable expressing her thoughts, feelings, and concerns without fear of judgment or criticism. Practice active listening when your daughter communicates with you, giving her your full attention and acknowledging her perspective.

Validate her feelings and experiences, even if you may not agree with them.

Model the behaviors and attitudes you want to see in your daughter, such as kindness, patience, responsibility, and resilience. Demonstrate effective problem-solving skills and coping strategies when faced with challenges. Teach your daughter how to resolve conflicts and disagreements constructively, emphasizing active listening, empathy, compromise, and negotiation. Encourage her to seek win-win solutions whenever possible.

Acknowledge and praise your daughter for following rules, meeting expectations, and demonstrating positive behavior. Offer rewards or incentives as motivators for desired behaviors, such as extra privileges or special treats. Focus on praising your daughter's efforts and improvements rather than just outcomes or achievements. Encourage her to persevere and continue making progress, even in the face of setbacks.

Fostering Self-Esteem and Resilience

Building self-esteem and resilience is essential for girls with attention-deficit/hyperactivity disorder (ADHD) to develop a strong sense of self-worth and the ability to bounce back from challenges.

Identify and celebrate your daughter's unique strengths, talents, and abilities. Encourage her to recognize her strengths and take pride in her accomplishments, no matter how small. Praise your daughter for her efforts and perseverance, emphasizing the value of hard work, determination, and resilience. Focus on her progress and growth, rather than just outcomes or achievements.

Teach your daughter to replace negative self-talk with positive affirmations and empowering statements. Encourage her to challenge self-doubt and negative beliefs about herself. Instill a growth mindset in your daughter by imparting the knowledge that skills and intelligence can be enhanced through hard work, education, and dedication. Motivate her to welcome challenges and perceive obstacles as chances for personal development.

Listen attentively to your daughter's thoughts, feelings, and experiences without judgment or criticism. Validate her emotions and provide empathy and understanding, even if you may not agree with her perspective. Offer words of encouragement, reassurance, and support to bolster your daughter's confidence and self-esteem. Assure her that you have faith in her capabilities and will always be by her side, offering unwavering support.

Teach your daughter effective coping skills and strategies for managing stress, anxiety, and frustration. Encourage her to practice relaxation techniques, mindfulness exercises, and deep breathing exercises. Help your daughter develop problem-solving skills by teaching her how to identify problems, brainstorm solutions, evaluate options, and make decisions independently. Encourage her to approach challenges with a positive attitude and a willingness to learn from mistakes.

Support your daughter in developing independence and autonomy by allowing her to make choices, take on responsibilities, and solve problems on her own. Offer guidance and support as needed, but encourage her to take ownership of her decisions and actions. Teach your daughter to advocate for herself by expressing her needs, asking for help when needed, and standing up for her rights and interests. Encourage her to communicate assertively and assert her boundaries in various situations.

Create a safe and nurturing home environment where your daughter feels accepted, valued, and supported. Foster open communication, mutual respect, and unconditional love within the family. Seek support from trusted friends, family members, or professionals if you need assistance in supporting your daughter's self-esteem and resilience. Connect with support groups or counseling services for additional guidance and resources.

Building a Support Network

Building a strong support network is essential for girls with attention-deficit/hyperactivity disorder (ADHD) to thrive and succeed in various aspects of their lives.

1. **Family Support:** Foster open and honest communication within your family. Encourage your daughter to express her thoughts, feelings, and

concerns, and listen attentively to her needs. Educate family members about ADHD and its impact on your daughter's life. Help them understand her strengths, challenges, and unique needs, fostering empathy and support.

2. **Educational Support:** Maintain open lines of communication with your daughter's teachers and school staff. Advocate for her needs and collaborate on strategies to support her academic success. Work with school officials to explore accommodations and support services that can help your daughter thrive in the classroom.

3. **Peer Support:** Encourage your daughter to build positive relationships with peers who understand and accept her. Facilitate opportunities for socialization through extracurricular activities, clubs, or community groups. Provide guidance and support to help your daughter develop social skills and navigate social interactions effectively. Role-play common social scenarios and coach her on communication and conflict resolution techniques.

4. **Professional Support:** Consult with healthcare professionals, such as

pediatricians, psychologists, or ADHD specialists, for guidance and support. They can offer insights into your daughter's condition and provide recommendations for treatment and management. Explore therapy options, such as cognitive-behavioral therapy (CBT) or social skills training, to help your daughter address challenges related to ADHD and develop coping strategies for managing symptoms.

5. **Community Resources**: Seek out local or online support groups for parents and families of children with ADHD. These groups can offer valuable insights, resources, and emotional support from others who understand your experiences. Explore community programs and resources designed to support children and families affected by ADHD. This may include educational workshops, recreational activities, or advocacy initiatives.

Connecting with Other Families and Support Groups

Connecting with other families and support groups can be incredibly beneficial for girls with attention-deficit/hyperactivity disorder (ADHD) and their parents. These connections provide valuable opportunities for sharing experiences, gaining insights, and accessing resources to support your daughter's journey.

- Online Support Communities: Explore online forums and discussion groups dedicated to ADHD and parenting. Websites like ADDitudeMag.com, Understood.org, and CHADD.org offer forums where parents can connect, ask questions, and share advice and experiences. Look for Facebook groups or Twitter chats focused on ADHD and parenting. These groups provide a platform for connecting with other families, sharing resources, and offering support in real-time.
- Local Support Groups: Inquire with local hospitals, community centers, or mental health organizations about support groups for families of children with ADHD. These groups may meet regularly to share experiences, learn from guest speakers, and access resources.
- Attend Parenting Workshops: Look for parenting workshops or seminars in

your area that focus on ADHD and related topics. These events can provide valuable information, support, and networking opportunities with other parents facing similar challenges.

- School-Based Support: Reach out to your daughter's school counselor or special education coordinator to inquire about support groups or parent networks for families of children with ADHD. These professionals may be able to provide referrals or facilitate connections with other families.
- Participate in Parent-Teacher Associations: Get involved in your daughter's school community by joining the Parent-Teacher Association (PTA) or similar parent groups. These organizations often host events and activities where parents can connect and support each other.
- Explore Therapy Options: Consider enrolling your daughter in group therapy or social skills groups specifically tailored for children with ADHD. These therapeutic settings provide a supportive environment for building social skills, self-esteem, and coping strategies.

- Seek Parent Coaching: Explore parent coaching programs or support services that specialize in ADHD and parenting. These programs offer guidance, strategies, and support to help parents navigate the challenges of raising a child with ADHD.
- Attend Virtual Meetups: Look for virtual meetups or webinars specifically designed for families of children with ADHD. These online events provide an opportunity to connect with other parents, share experiences, and access expert advice from the comfort of your home.
- Join Online Support Groups: Explore online support groups or video chat platforms where families of children with ADHD can connect and interact. These virtual support groups offer flexibility and convenience for busy parents to connect with others facing similar challenges.

Connecting with other families and support groups for girls with ADHD can provide invaluable support, understanding, and resources for both parents and children. Whether online or in-person, these connections offer opportunities to share experiences, gain insights, and access support from others who understand your journey.

Advocating for ADHD Awareness and Education

Advocating for ADHD awareness and education is crucial for promoting understanding, acceptance, and support for individuals affected by attention-deficit/hyperactivity disorder (ADHD), including girls.

Raise awareness by sharing your family's experiences with ADHD openly and honestly with friends, family members, and community members. Personal stories can help raise awareness and break down stigma surrounding ADHD.

Get involved in ADHD awareness campaigns and events in your community. This may include organizing or participating in walks, fundraisers, or educational seminars focused on ADHD.

Educate others by sharing accurate and up-to-date information about ADHD with educators, healthcare professionals, and community leaders. Provide resources, such as brochures, fact sheets, or online articles, to help educate others about the condition.

Advocate for training programs or workshops on ADHD for educators, healthcare providers, and other professionals who work with children. Provide opportunities for them to learn about ADHD symptoms, challenges, and best practices for support.

Advocate for policies and legislation that promote awareness, understanding, and support for individuals with ADHD. This may include advocating for increased funding for ADHD research, improved access to healthcare services, or better support in educational settings.

Join forces with local or national advocacy groups focused on ADHD to amplify your advocacy efforts. These groups may offer resources, guidance, and opportunities to advocate for policy changes at the local, state, or national level.

Advocate for inclusive environments that support the diverse needs of individuals with ADHD. Work with schools, workplaces, and community organizations to implement accommodations and supports that benefit individuals with ADHD.

Work with school administrators and educators to promote ADHD awareness and understanding in school settings. Advocate for policies and practices that support students with ADHD, such as flexible learning environments, positive behavior supports, and access to resources.

Organize community events, workshops, or support groups focused on ADHD awareness and education. Invite guest speakers, host panel discussions, or provide resources to help community members learn more about ADHD.

Partner with local organizations, businesses, or healthcare providers to raise awareness about ADHD in the community. Collaborate on events, initiatives, or outreach efforts to reach a broader audience.

Advocating for ADHD awareness and education is a powerful way to promote understanding, acceptance, and support for individuals affected by ADHD, including girls.

Understanding and Parenting Your Girl Child with ADHD

Chapter 6: Communication and Relationship Building

Effective communication and strong relationships are essential for supporting girls with attention-deficit hyperactivity disorder (ADHD) in navigating their challenges and achieving success. Here are some practical strategies for fostering communication and building positive relationships with girls with ADHD to help them thrive academically, socially, and emotionally.

1. Open and Honest Communication
Establish an environment where your daughter feels comfortable expressing her thoughts, feelings, and concerns without fear of judgment or criticism. Encourage open and honest communication by being approachable and non-judgmental.

Practice active listening by giving your daughter your full attention, maintaining eye contact, and responding with empathy and understanding.

2. Use Clear and Direct Language

Use clear, simple, and direct language when communicating with your daughter, avoiding vague or ambiguous terms. Provide specific instructions, expectations, and feedback to minimize misunderstandings.

Supplement verbal communication with visual aids such as charts, diagrams, or written instructions to enhance comprehension and retention for girls with ADHD who may benefit from visual cues.

3. Build Trust and Respect
Demonstrate honesty, reliability, and consistency in your words and actions to earn your daughter's trust. Follow through on promises and commitments, and be transparent about decisions that may affect her.

Respect your daughter's perspective, opinions, and autonomy, even if they differ from your own. Validate her feelings and experiences, and involve her in decision-making processes whenever possible.

4. Establish Boundaries and Expectations
Establish clear boundaries and expectations for behavior, responsibilities, and privileges

within the family. Communicate these boundaries calmly and consistently, and enforce them fairly and predictably.

Involve your daughter in the process of setting family rules and expectations, allowing her to contribute her input and perspective. This cooperative method fosters a feeling of responsibility and ownership.

5. Promote Positive Interactions and Conflict Resolution
Foster positive interactions and connections between family members by engaging in activities together, sharing experiences, and expressing appreciation and affection.

Teach your daughter effective conflict resolution skills, such as active listening, perspective-taking, compromise, and negotiation. Encourage her to communicate assertively and respectfully when resolving conflicts.

6. Celebrate Achievements and Growth
Celebrate your daughter's achievements, milestones, and progress, no matter how small. Offer praise, encouragement, and recognition for her efforts and accomplishments.

Emphasize the importance of continuous learning, growth, and improvement rather than perfection. Encourage your daughter to embrace challenges, learn from mistakes, and persevere in the face of setbacks.

Effective communication and positive relationships are essential for supporting girls with ADHD in reaching their full potential and thriving in all aspects of life. By fostering open and honest communication, using clear and direct language, building trust and respect, establishing boundaries and expectations, promoting positive interactions and conflict resolution, and celebrating achievements and growth, you can strengthen your relationship with your daughter and provide the support she needs to navigate the challenges of ADHD with confidence and resilience.

Effective Communication Strategies for Parents and Girls with ADHD

Effective communication is key to building strong relationships and supporting girls with attention-deficit hyperactivity disorder (ADHD) in managing their symptoms and achieving success.

- Use clear, straightforward language when communicating with your daughter, avoiding jargon or complicated explanations. Break down information into small, digestible chunks to facilitate understanding.
- Repeat important information or instructions to ensure your daughter grasps the message. Use repetition and reinforcement to help her retain information and follow through on tasks.
- Supplement verbal communication with visual aids such as charts, diagrams, or illustrations to reinforce key concepts and instructions. Visual aids can help girls with ADHD better comprehend information and remember tasks.
- Encourage your daughter to write down important information, instructions, or reminders in a notebook or planner. Writing things down can enhance memory and organization for girls with ADHD.
- Use a positive and supportive tone when communicating with your daughter, offering words of

encouragement and praise for her efforts and accomplishments. Focus on her strengths and progress, rather than dwelling on mistakes or challenges.

- Minimize criticism or negative feedback, which can undermine your daughter's confidence and self-esteem. Instead, provide constructive feedback and guidance in a supportive manner.
- Practice active listening by giving your daughter your full attention when she is speaking. It is important to sustain eye contact, nod occasionally, and offer verbal affirmations in order to demonstrate your engagement and attentiveness
- Reflect back what your daughter has said to ensure you understand her perspective correctly. Clarify any misunderstandings or uncertainties to promote clarity and mutual understanding.
- Encourage your daughter to share her thoughts, feelings, and ideas openly. Ask for her input and perspective on family decisions, activities, and plans to promote a sense of inclusion and empowerment.

- Set aside dedicated time each day to communicate and connect with your daughter without distractions. Use this time to check in, share updates, and discuss any concerns or issues she may be facing.
- Be fully present and engaged during communication time, putting aside electronic devices and other distractions. Show genuine interest in your daughter's thoughts and feelings, and be an active participant in the conversation.

Effective communication is essential for building strong relationships and supporting girls with ADHD in managing their symptoms and navigating daily challenges. By keeping communication clear and simple, providing visual and written support, maintaining a positive and supportive tone, practicing active listening, encouraging two-way communication, and setting aside quality time for communication, parents can foster understanding, cooperation, and mutual respect with their daughters with ADHD.

Strengthening Parent-Child Relationships

Building a strong parent-child relationship is crucial for supporting girls with attention-deficit/hyperactivity disorder (ADHD) in managing their symptoms and thriving in all aspects of life. Here are some ways you can use to strengthen the parent-child relationship specifically tailored to the challenges and needs of girls with ADHD.

1. Prioritize Quality Time Together: Set aside dedicated one-on-one time with your daughter on a regular basis. Use this time to engage in activities she enjoys, such as playing games, going for walks, or doing crafts together. Establish family rituals and traditions that foster connection and bonding, such as weekly movie nights, cooking together, or taking weekend outings. Consistent rituals provide a sense of security and predictability for girls with ADHD.

2. Practice Active Listening and Empathy: Practice active listening by giving your daughter your full attention when she speaks. Validate her feelings and experiences, showing empathy and understanding even if you may not agree with her perspective. Encourage

your daughter to express her emotions openly and honestly. Acknowledge her feelings, offering comfort and support when she is upset or struggling.

3. Foster Open Communication: Foster an open and non-judgmental environment where your daughter feels comfortable expressing her thoughts, feelings, and concerns. Encourage open communication by being approachable and receptive to her needs. Practice active listening, use clear and simple language, and provide visual aids or written instructions when necessary to facilitate understanding and communication.

4. Set Clear Boundaries and Expectations: Set clear rules and expectations for behavior, responsibilities, and privileges within the family. Communicate these boundaries calmly and consistently, and enforce them fairly and predictably. Involve your daughter in the process of setting family rules and expectations, allowing her to contribute her input and perspective.

5. Celebrate Achievements and Progress: Celebrate your daughter's efforts and accomplishments, no matter how small. Offer

praise, encouragement, and recognition for her hard work and perseverance. Emphasize the importance of continuous learning and growth, encouraging your daughter to embrace challenges and learn from mistakes.

6. Seek Professional Support and Guidance: Seek support from professionals such as therapists, counselors, or ADHD coaches who specialize in working with children and families affected by ADHD. These professionals can offer guidance, strategies, and resources to support your daughter and strengthen your parent-child relationship.

Connect with other parents of girls with ADHD through support groups or online forums. Sharing experiences, advice, and strategies with other parents can provide validation, encouragement, and solidarity.

Remember to be patient, compassionate, and understanding as you navigate the ups and downs of parenting a child with ADHD, focusing on nurturing a loving and supportive connection that will endure over time.

Navigating Challenging Behaviors with Empathy and Understanding

Girls with attention-deficit hyperactivity disorder (ADHD) may exhibit challenging behaviors that can test the patience and understanding of parents. Navigating these behaviors with empathy and understanding is crucial for maintaining a positive and supportive relationship while helping your daughter learn and grow. In this section, we will explore practical strategies for responding to challenging behaviors with empathy and understanding.

Educate yourself about the symptoms and characteristics of ADHD, including impulsivity, hyperactivity, and inattention. Recognize that your daughter's challenging behaviors may be manifestations of her ADHD rather than deliberate defiance.

Identify potential triggers or stressors that may contribute to your daughter's challenging behaviors, such as sensory sensitivities, academic difficulties, or social stressors. Understanding these triggers can help you respond with empathy and compassion.

Maintain a calm and composed demeanor when responding to your daughter's challenging behaviors. Avoid reacting impulsively or emotionally, as this can escalate the situation and make it more difficult to resolve.

Recognize that change takes time, and your daughter may need patience and support as she learns to manage her behaviors. Respond to setbacks with patience and understanding, focusing on progress rather than perfection.

Demonstrate empathy and understanding toward your daughter's feelings and experiences, even when her behaviors are challenging. Let her know that you understand and care about her struggles, and that you are there to support her.

Acknowledge your daughter's emotions and feelings, even if you may not agree with her behavior. Let her know that it's okay to feel frustrated, angry, or upset, and offer comfort and support as she navigates her emotions.

Reinforce positive behaviors and accomplishments with praise, encouragement, and rewards. Focus on the behaviors you want to see more of, rather than dwelling on the negative.

Offer words of encouragement and support to your daughter, reminding her that you believe in her abilities and strengths. Encourage her to keep trying and persevering, even when faced with challenges.

Include your daughter in the process of problem-solving and finding solutions to her challenging behaviors. Encourage her to brainstorm ideas and strategies for managing her impulses and emotions.

Provide guidance and support as your daughter explores different coping strategies and techniques. Offer suggestions and resources that may help her better understand and regulate her emotions and behaviors.

If your daughter's challenging behaviors persist or significantly impact her daily functioning, consider seeking support from mental health professionals, such as therapists or behavioral specialists. They can offer additional strategies and interventions tailored to your daughter's needs.

Understanding and Parenting Your Girl Child with ADHD

Join support groups or online communities for parents of children with ADHD. Sharing experiences and resources with other parents can provide valuable insights and support as you navigate challenging behaviors together.

Navigating challenging behaviors with empathy and understanding is essential for maintaining a positive and supportive relationship with your daughter with ADHD.

Chapter 7: Developing Coping Skills and Self-Regulation

Developing effective coping skills and self-regulation strategies is crucial for girls with attention-deficit/hyperactivity disorder (ADHD) to manage their symptoms, navigate challenges, and thrive in various aspects of life. Let's explore practical techniques and approaches to help girls with ADHD develop coping skills and enhance self-regulation.

1. Mindfulness and Relaxation Techniques: Teach your daughter deep breathing exercises to help her calm her mind and body when feeling overwhelmed or anxious. Practice together and encourage her to use this technique whenever needed. Introduce mindfulness practices, such as mindful breathing or body scans, to help your daughter become more aware of her thoughts, emotions, and bodily sensations. Mindfulness can enhance self-regulation and emotional resilience.

2. Organization and Time Management Strategies: Encourage your daughter to use

planners, calendars, or digital apps to keep track of assignments, appointments, and responsibilities. Help her develop a system for prioritizing tasks and managing her time effectively. Teach your daughter to break large tasks or projects into smaller, more manageable steps. This approach can help reduce feelings of overwhelm and increase her sense of accomplishment.

3. Problem-Solving and Decision-Making Skills: Encourage your daughter to identify the specific problem or challenge she is facing. Help her articulate the problem clearly and objectively to gain a better understanding of the situation. Guide your daughter through the process of brainstorming potential solutions to the problem. Encourage creativity and flexibility in generating ideas, and explore both short-term and long-term solutions.

4. Emotional Regulation Strategies: Help your daughter identify common triggers for emotional dysregulation, such as frustration, criticism, or sensory overload. Once identified, work together to develop strategies for managing these triggers. Teach your daughter to challenge negative thoughts and replace them with positive affirmations or coping

statements. Encourage her to practice self-compassion and kindness toward herself.

5. Social Skills and Conflict Resolution Techniques: Engage in role-playing activities with your daughter to practice social skills and conflict resolution techniques. Role-play common social situations or conflicts she may encounter, and explore different ways to respond effectively. Teach your daughter active listening skills, such as maintaining eye contact, nodding, and paraphrasing what others say. Help her learn to empathize with others' perspectives and communicate assertively.

6. Seeking Support and Assistance: Emphasize the importance of seeking support and assistance when needed. Teach your daughter to recognize when she needs help and to reach out to trusted adults, friends, or professionals for support. Familiarize yourself with available resources and support services for girls with ADHD, such as therapy, counseling, or ADHD coaching. Encourage your daughter to explore these resources as needed.

Teaching Emotional Regulation and Stress Management Techniques

Emotional regulation and stress management are essential skills for girls with attention-deficit hyperactivity disorder (ADHD) to navigate the ups and downs of life effectively.

Teach your daughter to identify and label her emotions accurately. Encourage her to recognize the physical sensations and thoughts associated with different emotions, such as anger, frustration, or anxiety. Expand your daughter's emotional vocabulary by introducing new words to describe various feelings. Help her articulate her emotions using descriptive language, such as "I feel disappointed" or "I'm experiencing overwhelm."

Guide your daughter through simple breathing exercises to help her become more mindful of her breath and its calming effect on her body. Practice slow, deep breathing together, focusing on the sensation of the breath entering and leaving the body. Lead your daughter through a body scan meditation, where she systematically focuses her attention on different parts of her body, noticing any tension or discomfort.

Teach your daughter to challenge negative thoughts and replace them with positive affirmations or coping statements. Encourage her to reframe negative situations in a more optimistic light. Explore different stress reduction techniques with your daughter, such as progressive muscle relaxation, guided imagery, or visualization exercises. Help her find activities that promote relaxation and calmness, such as listening to music, drawing, or spending time in nature.

Work with your daughter to identify common triggers for stress or emotional dysregulation. Help her recognize patterns in her behavior and emotions, and brainstorm strategies for managing these triggers proactively. Guide your daughter through the process of problem-solving, encouraging her to generate potential solutions to the challenges she faces. Explore the pros and cons of each solution and help her select the most effective course of action.

Normalize the idea of seeking support and assistance when needed. Let your daughter know that it's okay to ask for help from trusted adults, friends, or professionals when she's feeling overwhelmed or struggling to cope.

Familiarize yourself and your daughter with available resources and support services for managing stress and emotions, such as therapy, support groups, or online forums. Encourage her to reach out for help when necessary.

Building Executive Functioning Skills

Executive functioning skills are crucial for success in academics, relationships, and daily life tasks. Girls with attention-deficit/hyperactivity disorder (ADHD) often struggle with executive functioning deficits, but with targeted support and strategies, they can develop these essential skills. In this section, we will explore practical techniques to help girls with ADHD build executive functioning skills.

1. Organization and Planning
Encourage your daughter to use visual aids such as calendars, planners, or to-do lists to organize her tasks and activities. Help her

break down large tasks into smaller, more manageable steps. Create consistent routines and schedules for your daughter to follow, including designated times for homework, chores, and extracurricular activities. Consistent routines provide structure and predictability, which can support executive functioning.

2. Time Management
Teach your daughter to use time-blocking techniques to allocate specific blocks of time for different tasks or activities. It is advisable to prompt her to make estimations on the duration of each task and plan her schedule accordingly. Introduce the use of timers or alarms to help your daughter stay on track and manage her time effectively. Set timers for tasks or transitions to help her stay focused and accountable.

3. Impulse Control
Encourage your daughter to pause and reflect before acting impulsively. Teach her to take a moment to consider the consequences of her actions and whether they align with her goals and values. Help your daughter develop self-discipline by setting clear boundaries and expectations. Provide positive reinforcement

and praise when she demonstrates self-control and restraint.

4. Flexibility and Adaptability

Teach your daughter problem-solving skills to help her navigate unexpected challenges or changes in plans. Encourage her to brainstorm alternative solutions and consider different perspectives. Help your daughter develop coping strategies for dealing with setbacks or failures. Encourage her to adopt a growth mindset and view challenges as opportunities for learning and growth.

5. Working Memory

Break down information into smaller chunks to make it easier for your daughter to process and remember. Encourage her to use mnemonic devices or visualization techniques to aid memory retention. Review important information frequently and encourage your daughter to repeat key concepts or instructions to reinforce learning. Provide opportunities for practice and repetition to strengthen working memory skills.

6. Seeking Support and Assistance

Normalize the idea of seeking support and assistance when needed. Let your daughter know that it's okay to ask for help from teachers, parents, or peers when she's struggling with executive functioning tasks. Familiarize yourself and your daughter with available resources and support services for developing executive functioning skills, such as educational programs, tutoring, or executive functioning coaches.

By implementing these strategies and providing ongoing support, you can help your daughter with ADHD build essential executive functioning skills that will serve her well in school, relationships, and life. Remember to be patient, consistent, and encouraging as she develops and refines these skills, and celebrate her progress along the way.

Encouraging Independence and Problem-Solving Abilities

Encouraging independence and fostering problem-solving abilities are essential for girls with attention-deficit hyperactivity disorder (ADHD) to navigate the challenges of daily life effectively.

To do this gradually increase your daughter's responsibilities and independence over time, starting with small tasks and gradually expanding to more complex ones. Provide guidance and support as needed, but encourage her to take ownership of her actions.

Give your daughter opportunities to make decisions and choices independently, such as selecting her own clothing, planning meals, or managing her time. Offer guidance and feedback, but allow her to experience the consequences of her decisions.

Let your daughter think critically and analytically about problems or challenges she encounters. Ask open-ended questions to stimulate her thinking and help her explore different perspectives. Teach your daughter to break down problems or tasks into smaller, more manageable steps.

Encourage her to brainstorm potential solutions and consider the pros and cons of each option.. Help your daughter evaluate the potential outcomes and consequences of different choices before making a decision. Encourage her to consider both short-term and long-term consequences, as well as her own values and priorities.

Provide opportunities for your daughter to practice making choices and decisions in various contexts, such as choosing extracurricular activities, setting personal goals, or resolving conflicts with friends.

Let your daughter view mistakes and setbacks as opportunities for growth and learning rather than failures. Help her develop resilience by reframing challenges as temporary obstacles that she can overcome with effort and perseverance.

Offer emotional support and encouragement when your daughter faces difficulties or setbacks. Acknowledge her emotions and encounters, and provide reassurance that obstacles are an inherent aspect of the educational journey. Let your daughter take initiative and seek out opportunities for learning and growth on her own.

Support her interests and passions, and provide resources and guidance to help her pursue them. Teach your daughter to be resourceful and adaptable in solving problems and overcoming obstacles. Encourage her to use her creativity and resourcefulness to find innovative solutions to challenges she encounters.

Foster a collaborative and supportive environment where your daughter feels comfortable seeking help and support from others when needed. Encourage her to collaborate with peers, teachers, or family members to solve problems and achieve goals.

Familiarize your daughter with available resources and support services that can assist her in developing independence and problem-solving skills, such as mentorship programs, tutoring, or community organizations.

Encourage her to take initiative, embrace challenges, and seek out opportunities for growth and learning. Provide ongoing support, guidance, and encouragement as she navigates the journey toward independence, and celebrate her accomplishments along the way. With your support and encouragement, she can overcome obstacles and thrive in all aspects of her life.

Chapter 8: Celebrating Strengths and Talents

Girls with attention-deficit hyperactivity disorder (ADHD) possess unique strengths, talents, and qualities that deserve recognition and celebration.

Encourage your daughter to reflect on her own strengths, talents, and interests. Help her identify areas where she excels, whether it's in academics, sports, creative pursuits, or interpersonal skills. Celebrate your daughter's unique qualities and characteristics that make her who she is. Whether it's her creativity, empathy, sense of humor, or determination, let her know that her individuality is something to be celebrated.

Encourage your daughter to explore her passions and interests, whether it's art, music, science, or athletics. Provide opportunities for her to pursue these interests through classes, clubs, or extracurricular activities. Provide resources and guidance to help your daughter further develop her talents and interests. Whether it's enrolling her in a painting class, supporting her in learning a musical instrument, or providing access to books and materials related to her interests, show your support for her pursuits.

Celebrate your daughter's achievements and milestones, no matter how small. Whether it's earning a good grade on a test, completing a challenging project, or mastering a new skill, acknowledge her efforts and accomplishments. Offer specific and genuine praise for your daughter's strengths and efforts. Focus on her strengths and progress rather than dwelling on shortcomings or mistakes.

Provide opportunities for your daughter to take on leadership roles and responsibilities. Whether it's leading a group project at school, organizing a community service initiative, or mentoring younger children, encourage her to step into leadership positions where she can use her strengths and talents to make a positive impact. Support your daughter in taking initiative and pursuing her goals and aspirations.

Encourage her to set goals for herself and take proactive steps toward achieving them. Offer guidance and encouragement as she navigates the path toward her dreams.

Understanding and Parenting Your Girl Child with ADHD

Emphasize the importance of diversity and individuality, both within your family and in the broader community. Teach your daughter to appreciate and respect the unique strengths and talents of others, fostering a culture of acceptance and inclusivity.

Create an environment where your daughter feels free to express herself authentically and creatively. Whether it's through art, writing, music, or other forms of self-expression, encourage her to share her thoughts, ideas, and talents with the world. Celebrating strengths and talents in girls with ADHD is essential for fostering confidence, resilience, and self-esteem.

By acknowledging and nurturing their unique qualities, interests, and achievements, you empower them to embrace their individuality and pursue their dreams with confidence and determination. Encourage your daughter to recognize her strengths, pursue her passions, and believe in herself, knowing that her talents are valuable and worthy of celebration. With your support and encouragement, she can overcome challenges and shine brightly in all aspects of her life.

Apart from encouraging them to nurture their abilities, you should be able to recognise their gifts. It's essential to recognize and celebrate the unique gifts and talents of girls with ADHD, as they have much to offer the world.

Recognizing the Unique Gifts of Girls with ADHD

Girls with attention-deficit/hyperactivity disorder (ADHD) possess a wealth of unique gifts, talents, and strengths that often go unrecognized. In this section, we will explore the distinctive qualities and contributions of girls with ADHD and the importance of acknowledging and celebrating their individuality.

1. **Creativity and Innovation:** Girls with ADHD often demonstrate remarkable creativity and innovation. Their ability to think outside the box and see things from unconventional perspectives can lead to breakthrough ideas and solutions. Many girls with ADHD excel in creative pursuits such as art, music, writing, and drama. Their vivid imagination and boundless energy fuel their artistic endeavors, producing original and expressive works.

2. **Hyperfocus and Intense Passion:** While ADHD is commonly associated with distractibility, girls with ADHD also have the ability to hyperfocus intensely on tasks that capture their interest. When engaged in activities they enjoy, they can exhibit remarkable concentration and productivity. Girls with ADHD often demonstrate intense passion and enthusiasm for their interests and hobbies. Whether it's a favorite subject in school, a sport, or a creative project, they dive into their passions wholeheartedly, often achieving impressive results.

3. **Keen Observational Skills:** Despite challenges with sustained attention, girls with ADHD often possess keen observational skills. They notice details that others may overlook and can be highly perceptive in social situations, picking up on subtle cues and nuances. Girls with ADHD are naturally curious and eager to explore the world around them. Their inquisitive nature leads them to ask probing questions, seek out new experiences, and pursue knowledge with enthusiasm.

4. **Empathy and Compassion:** Contrary to the stereotype of ADHD as a purely hyperactive or impulsive condition, girls with ADHD often

demonstrate a high degree of empathy and emotional sensitivity. They are attuned to others' feelings and are quick to offer support and compassion.

Girls with ADHD have a strong sense of fairness and justice, and they are often passionate advocates for causes they believe in. They have a deep-seated desire to make the world a better place and are willing to speak up for what they believe is right.

5. **Resilience and Determination:** Despite facing numerous challenges associated with ADHD, girls with this condition demonstrate remarkable resilience and determination. They persevere in the face of setbacks, learn from their mistakes, and bounce back stronger than ever. Girls with ADHD possess an unwavering spirit and zest for life that is infectious. Their boundless energy and optimism inspire those around them, and they approach life with a sense of adventure and enthusiasm.

By acknowledging their creativity, passion, empathy, resilience, and other strengths, we can empower them to embrace their individuality and thrive in all aspects of life.

Apart from these, girls with ADHD have many interests and hobbies you should help them cultivate.

Cultivating Interests and Hobbies

Cultivating interests and hobbies plays a crucial role in the development and well-being of girls with attention-deficit/hyperactivity disorder (ADHD). Engaging in activities they enjoy can help them channel their energy, build confidence, and develop important skills. In this section, we will explore strategies for identifying and nurturing interests and hobbies in girls with ADHD.

→ Introduce your daughter to a variety of activities and interests to help her discover what she enjoys. Take her to museums, concerts, sports events, or art classes to expose her to different hobbies and pursuits.

→ Pay attention to your daughter's natural inclinations and preferences. Notice what activities she shows interest in and encourage her to explore them further.

→ Encourage your daughter to pursue a range of interests, from sports and outdoor activities to creative pursuits like art, music, and writing. Celebrate her diverse interests and support her in exploring different hobbies.

→ Offer resources and opportunities to support your daughter's interests, such as enrolling her in classes or workshops, providing access to materials and equipment, or connecting her with mentors in her areas of interest.

→ Cultivate an environment that fosters curiosity and exploration. Encourage your daughter to ask questions, seek out new experiences, and pursue her interests with enthusiasm.

→ Provide positive reinforcement and encouragement as your daughter explores new hobbies and interests. Celebrate her efforts and accomplishments, and let her know that you support her in pursuing her passions.

→ Encourage regular practice and skill development in your daughter's chosen hobbies. Set aside time for her to engage in her interests, and provide opportunities for her to refine her skills and learn new techniques.

→ Help your daughter set achievable goals related to her hobbies, whether it's mastering a new song on the guitar, completing a challenging puzzle, or improving her soccer skills. Break larger goals into smaller, more manageable steps to maintain motivation and progress.

→ Recognize and celebrate your daughter's efforts and progress in her hobbies and interests. Focus on her growth and development rather than solely on outcomes, and let her know that you're proud of her dedication and hard work.

→ Provide opportunities for your daughter to share her interests and accomplishments with others. Whether it's performing in a recital, displaying artwork, or participating in a team sport, encourage her to share her talents and passions with pride.

By cultivating her interests and hobbies, you can help your daughter with ADHD discover her passions, build confidence, and develop important skills that will benefit her throughout life.

Here are more ways to help your daughter with her growth mindset.

Fostering a Growth Mindset and Resilience

Fostering a growth mindset and resilience is crucial for girls with attention-deficit hyperactivity disorder (ADHD) to navigate the challenges they face and thrive in all aspects of life.

1. Encourage your daughter to focus on effort rather than innate ability. Teach her that intelligence and abilities can be developed through hard work, practice, and perseverance. Help your daughter understand that making mistakes is a natural part of the learning process. Emphasize the importance of learning from mistakes, bouncing back, and trying again.
2. Help your daughter challenge negative self-talk and limiting beliefs. Encourage her to reframe negative thoughts and replace them with positive affirmations and empowering statements. Encourage your daughter to set realistic goals and expectations for herself.
3. Serve as a role model for resilience by demonstrating resilience in your own life. Share stories of overcoming

challenges and setbacks, and highlight the importance of perseverance and determination. Equip your daughter with coping strategies to help her navigate adversity and setbacks. Teach her techniques for managing stress, regulating emotions, and problem-solving effectively.

4. Recognize and celebrate your daughter's efforts and progress, regardless of the outcome. Focus on the process rather than solely on outcomes, and praise her for her hard work, determination, and resilience. Point out instances where your daughter has demonstrated growth and improvement. Help her see how her efforts and perseverance have led to positive outcomes and personal growth.

5. Let your daughter know that you are there to support her unconditionally, no matter what challenges she faces. Provide a safe and nurturing environment where she feels comfortable expressing herself and seeking help when needed. Offer words of encouragement and reassurance to bolster your daughter's confidence and self-esteem. Remind her of her

strengths, talents, and past successes, and encourage her to believe in herself.

By fostering a growth mindset and resilience in girls with ADHD, you empower them to overcome obstacles, bounce back from setbacks, and achieve their full potential. Encourage a positive mindset, promote a can-do attitude, build resilience, celebrate effort and progress, and provide unconditional support and encouragement. With your guidance and support, your daughter can develop the resilience and mindset needed to thrive in the face of adversity and succeed in all areas of life.

Conclusion

Looking ahead, parenting a girl with ADHD is a journey filled with challenges, triumphs, and growth for both parent and child alike. As we continue on this journey, it's essential to remember that every girl with ADHD is unique, with her own strengths, weaknesses, and potential.

Embracing this journey means recognizing that there will be ups and downs along the way, but also understanding that with patience, perseverance, and support, our daughters can overcome obstacles and thrive. It means celebrating their achievements, no matter how small, and supporting them through setbacks and struggles.

As parents, it's crucial to continue educating ourselves about ADHD, staying informed about the latest research and treatment options, and advocating for our daughters' needs. It's about building a strong support network of professionals, friends, and family members who understand and accept our daughters for who they are.

It's also about fostering a positive mindset and resilience in both ourselves and our daughters, helping them develop coping skills, self-regulation techniques, and a strong sense of self-worth. It's about teaching them to embrace their strengths and talents, while also acknowledging and addressing their challenges.

Above all, it's about loving our daughters unconditionally, supporting them wholeheartedly, and believing in their potential to achieve greatness. Parenting a girl with ADHD may not always be easy, but it's a journey filled with love, learning, and endless possibilities. And with dedication, patience, and a whole lot of love, we can navigate this journey together and help our daughters soar.

In conclusion, understanding and parenting girls with ADHD requires a multifaceted approach that encompasses education, support, and advocacy. Throughout this book, we have explored the unique challenges and strengths of girls with ADHD, as well as strategies for effectively supporting them in various aspects of their lives.

We began by discussing the importance of recognizing ADHD in girls, as well as the factors that contribute to the underdiagnosis and misdiagnosis of ADHD in this population. We then delved into the neurobiology of ADHD, gender differences in presentation, and common signs and symptoms to look out for.

Next, we explored the impact of ADHD on girls across developmental stages, including academic challenges, social and emotional implications, and coping mechanisms. We also discussed the importance of early intervention and the role of parents in advocating for their child's needs in school and community settings.

Throughout the book, I emphasized the importance of fostering a supportive environment, building a strong support network, and seeking professional guidance and resources. I highlighted the value of connecting with other families and support groups, advocating for ADHD awareness and education, and promoting ADHD-friendly environments in schools and communities.

Armed with all this knowledge and determination, Maya and her family embarked on a journey of understanding and acceptance. They learned about the unique challenges faced by individuals with ADHD and discovered strategies to manage symptoms effectively. Maya began therapy sessions to work on executive functioning skills and received accommodations at school to support her learning needs.

As Maya learned more about her ADHD, she started to embrace her strengths and talents. She realized that her assertiveness and leadership skills were not flaws but valuable assets. With the encouragement of her family and teachers, Maya channeled her energy into positive outlets, such as organizing charity events and mentoring younger students.

Over time, Maya's confidence soared, and the label of "bossy" or "little madam" as she nicknamed, no longer held power over her. Instead, Maya was celebrated for her leadership abilities and admired for her resilience in the face of adversity. She became a role model for other children with ADHD, showing them that they, too, could overcome obstacles and achieve their dreams.

As Maya looked back on her journey, she realized that her ADHD was not a limitation but a source of strength. She had learned to embrace her uniqueness and advocate for herself, paving the way for a bright and promising future.

And so, Maya's story serves as a reminder that with patience, understanding, and support, every child has the potential to thrive, regardless of their challenges.

In the end, my goal is to empower you as a parent with the knowledge, resources, and support you need to help your daughters with ADHD thrive. Just like Maya and her parents used the knowledge in this book to help their daughter reach her full potential and lead a fulfilling life.

Final Words of Encouragement and Inspiration

In closing, I want to let you know that you are not alone on this journey. While parenting a girl with ADHD may come with its unique set of challenges, remember that you are not alone. There is a community of parents, caregivers, and professionals who understand and support you every step of the way.

Believe in your daughter's potential. Your daughter is capable of achieving incredible things, regardless of the challenges she may face. Believe in her strengths, talents, and abilities, and encourage her to pursue her passions with confidence and determination.

Celebrate every success, no matter how small. Every milestone, achievement, and moment of progress is worth celebrating. Take the time to acknowledge and celebrate your daughter's accomplishments, no matter how small they may seem.

Practice self-care and compassion. Remember to take care of yourself and prioritize your own well-being. Parenting a child with ADHD can be exhausting and overwhelming at times, so be sure to practice self-care and show yourself compassion along the way.

Keep learning and growing. Stay informed about ADHD and continue to educate yourself about the latest research, treatments, and strategies for supporting your daughter. Never stop learning and growing as a parent and advocate.

Above all, remember that you are doing the best you can for your daughter, and that is more than enough. Your love, dedication, and unwavering support make all the difference in her life. Keep believing in her, keep advocating for her, and never underestimate the incredible impact you have as her parent or caregiver.

You've got this, and your daughter is lucky to have you by her side on this journey. Keep shining brightly, and never forget the incredible potential that lies within your daughter and within yourself.

Additional Resources

"*Smart but Scattered: The Revolutionary 'Executive Skills' Approach to Helping Kids Reach Their Potential*" by Peg Dawson and Richard Guare
https://www.ncbi.nlm.nih.gov/pmc/articles/PMC3829464/

"*The Survival Guide for Kids with ADHD*" by John F. Taylor
https://www.adhdevidence.org/

"*Taking Charge of ADHD: The Complete, Authoritative Guide for Parents*" by Russell A. Barkley

CHADD (Children and Adults with Attention-Deficit/Hyperactivity Disorder): Offers resources, support groups, and educational materials for individuals with ADHD and their families. Website: chadd.org

ADDitude Magazine: Provides articles, webinars, and expert advice on ADHD-related topics for parents, caregivers, and individuals with ADHD. Website: additudemag.com

Understood: Offers resources and support for parents of children with learning and attention issues, including ADHD. Website: understood.org

ADHD Parent Support Group (Facebook Group): A supportive community for parents of children with ADHD to connect, share experiences, and offer advice. Website: facebook.com/groups/ADHDParentSupportGroup/

Reddit ADHD Community: An online forum where individuals with ADHD, parents, and caregivers can ask questions, share stories, and offer support to one another. Website: reddit.com/r/ADHD/

Professional Organizations:

American Academy of Child and Adolescent Psychiatry (AACAP): Provides resources and information on ADHD, including treatment options and finding mental health professionals. Website: aacap.org

American Psychological Association (APA): Offers information on ADHD, including diagnosis, treatment, and finding a psychologist. Website: apa.org

Local Support Groups:

Check with local hospitals, mental health centers, or community organizations to inquire about support groups for parents of children with ADHD in your area. These groups can provide valuable opportunities for in-person support and networking.

Bonus

The bonus attached to this book is a daily/weekly planner or checklist that your girl can use to plan her days.

It's a complete one month planner. Enjoy!

MY PLANNER

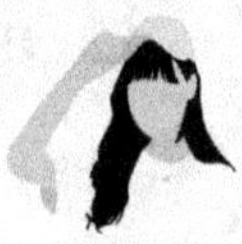

NAME

AGE

MONTHLY GOALS

PRIORITIES

NOTES

REMINDER

Weekly Planner

MONDAY — Date: _____
- ○
- ○
- ○
- ○

TUESDAY — Date: _____
- ○
- ○
- ○
- ○

WEDNESDAY — Date: _____
- ○
- ○
- ○
- ○

THURSDAY — Date: _____
- ○
- ○
- ○
- ○

FRIDAY — Date: _____
- ○
- ○
- ○
- ○

SATURDAY — Date: _____
- ○
- ○
- ○
- ○

SUNDAY — Date: _____
- ○
- ○
- ○
- ○

PRIORITIES
- ○
- ○
- ○
- ○
- ○

REMINDER

NEXT WEEK

Notes

Weekly Planner

PRIORITIES

MONDAY   Date: _____

○ _______________________
○ _______________________
○ _______________________
○ _______________________

TUESDAY   Date: _____

○ _______________________
○ _______________________
○ _______________________
○ _______________________

WEDNESDAY   Date: _____

○ _______________________
○ _______________________
○ _______________________
○ _______________________

THURSDAY   Date: _____

○ _______________________
○ _______________________
○ _______________________
○ _______________________

FRIDAY   Date: _____

○ _______________________
○ _______________________
○ _______________________
○ _______________________

SATURDAY   Date: _____

○ _______________________
○ _______________________
○ _______________________
○ _______________________

SUNDAY   Date: _____

○ _______________________
○ _______________________
○ _______________________
○ _______________________

PRIORITIES

○ _______________________
○ _______________________
○ _______________________
○ _______________________
○ _______________________

REMINDER

NEXT WEEK

Notes

Weekly Planner

PRIORITIES

MONDAY Date: ____

TUESDAY Date: ____

WEDNESDAY Date: ____

REMINDER

THURSDAY Date: ____

NEXT WEEK

FRIDAY Date: ____

Notes

SATURDAY Date: ____

SUNDAY Date: ____

Weekly Planner

MONDAY Date: ______

TUESDAY Date: ______

WEDNESDAY Date: ______

THURSDAY Date: ______

FRIDAY Date: ______

SATURDAY Date: ______

SUNDAY Date: ______

PRIORITIES

REMINDER

NEXT WEEK

Notes

www.ingramcontent.com/pod-product-compliance
Lightning Source LLC
Chambersburg PA
CBHW061640250726
48659CB00004B/1319